Preventing AIDS

A Guide to Effective Education for the Prevention of HIV Infection

Printed and bound in the United States of America.

American Public Health Association
1015 Fifteenth Street, NW
Washington, DC 20005

William H. McBeath, MD, MPH
Executive Director

The opinions expressed in the publication are the author's and do not necessarily represent the views or official policies of the Association.

ISBN 0-87553-166-0

Design and Typography: Page Designs Unlimited, Bethesda, Maryland
Printing and Binding: Sauls Lithograph, Washington, D.C.

Preventing AIDS

A Guide to Effective Education for the Prevention of HIV Infection

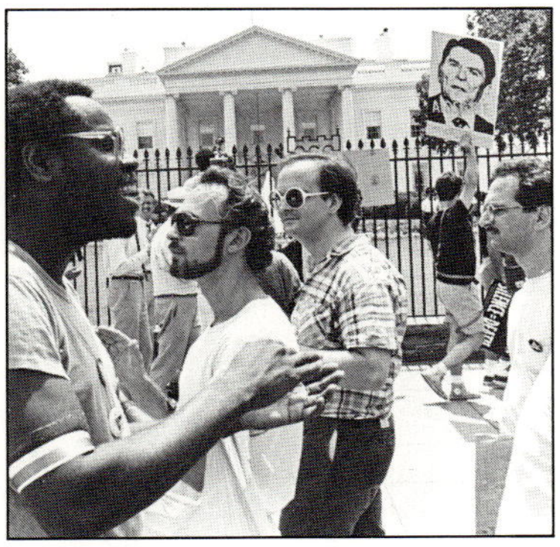

by Nicholas Freudenberg, DrPH

Professor and Director

Program in Community Health Education

Hunter College/CUNY

AMERICAN PUBLIC HEALTH ASSOCIATION

1015 Fifteenth Street, NW, Suite 300, Washington, DC 20005

(202) 789-5600

C O N T E N T S

Section 1. Planning AIDS Education Programs

Section 2. Reaching Out: How To Educate Specific Population Groups About AIDS

Introduction and Acknowledgments

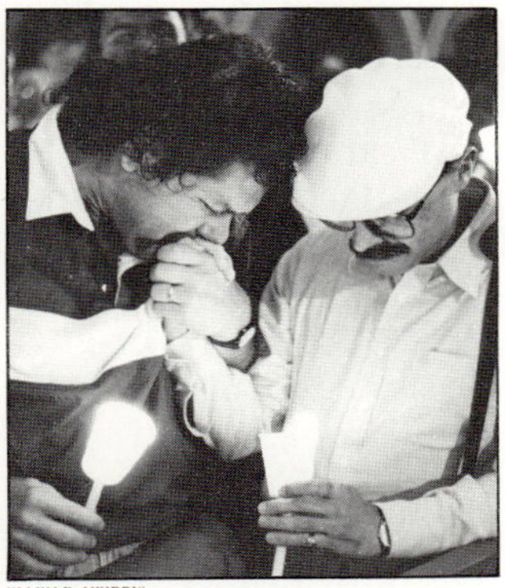

ELLEN B. NEIPRIS

While nearly everyone agrees that education is the most effective tool for controlling the acquired immune deficiency syndrome (AIDS) epidemic, debate continues on the most effective content and methods of education. Some of this debate is political: Should condoms be advertised on television? Should all children receive sex education in their schools? Should intravenous (IV) drug users learn how to sterilize their needles? Other controversies are more pedagogical: What is the best way to reach IV drug users, African-American and Latino youth, and women in the child-bearing years? How can one judge whether an education program has been successful?

Preventing AIDS *seeks to help all those involved in the struggle to control AIDS to develop more effective education programs. It summarizes what we have learned from seven years of experience educating people about AIDS. Using case histories of successful and unsuccessful efforts, it provides readers with a framework for making decisions about AIDS education. The guide includes information on both the social and political forces that influence AIDS educators, and practical advice on how to assess a population's needs, develop education* materials, build coalitions, and evaluate program effectiveness. Because its emphasis is on *prevention,* this guide does not discuss the important educational work being carried out to educate and support people who have AIDS. Readers seeking more information on this topic should consult the "Resources" section at the end of the guide.

Preventing AIDS is for health educators, nurses, community organizers, activists, teachers, health department officials—anyone involved in teaching the public about AIDS. It seeks to help public health practitioners to develop more effective AIDS prevention programs. Because many leaders of AIDS prevention programs have not had professional training in health education or AIDS, this guide provides a supplement to the on-the-job experience that AIDS prevention workers have accumulated.

To prepare this publication, more than 130 AIDS educators around the country were interviewed. Their names are listed beginning on page xi. The publication reflects their collective experiences and wisdom. They gave up precious time from fighting the epidemic to be interviewed because they wanted others to learn from their successes and failures. We also reviewed AIDS education materials from programs around the country and read the growing body of lay and professional articles on AIDS education. This guide reflects a synthesis of these sources.

In the future, AIDS educators will have the benefit of rigorous evaluation studies that are now being conducted. For the present, however, this review of program descriptions and educators' perceptions of their work can provide valuable guidance for those who need to plan and carry out AIDS education programs now.

The first section of *Preventing AIDS* describes the process for planning AIDS education. Chapter 1 analyzes the social and political context of AIDS education. Because the epidemic of human immunodeficiency virus (HIV) infection is so clearly embedded in broader social forces, AIDS educators must understand how these currents can both shape their work and be shaped in turn by the educators.

Chapter 2 describes how these social factors block or facilitate building support for AIDS prevention programs in agencies and communities and seeks to help AIDS educators generate the ongoing support they need if their goals are to be achieved.

Chapter 3 places the challenges of AIDS education within the larger discipline of health education. By understanding the methods that health educators use to plan, implement, and evaluate their work, AIDS educators can ground their activities in a conceptual framework.

Chapter 4 describes specific strategies that AIDS educators have used to achieve their goals. These include written materials, telephone hotlines, HIV antibody counseling and testing, mass media, training volunteers and professionals, condom campaigns, and community education. Each section discusses some of the advantages and limitations of the strategy and provides specific examples of the problems and solutions AIDS educators have encountered.

In Section II, the special needs and experiences of AIDS educators working with specific populations are described. Chapters are presented on gay and bisexual men, IV drug users, African-Americans and Latinos,* youth, women, workers, prisoners, people with hemophilia, homeless people, and disabled people. An important theme in Section II and throughout the guide is that everyone can play a role in AIDS prevention, no matter what their personal risk status. By synthesizing the

* In this guide, the designations African-American and Black are used interchangeably to describe Americans who themselves or whose ancestors came to the United States or the Caribbean region from Africa. Latino describes peoples who themselves or whose ancestors came to the United States from Central or South America or Caribbean countries where Spanish is the primary language. See Chapter 7 for further discussion of these terms.

experiences, problems, and recommendations of AIDS educators working with each of various populations, the guide seeks to help practitioners and planners anticipate the issues they will encounter and plan thoughtful responses.

Finally, a "Resources" section lists publications and organizations that readers can turn to for more information.

Readers can use the guide in different ways. Faced with a specific task, some may want to read the relevant section. An educator preparing a new program for inmates, for example, may read the prison section; or a health department official developing an HIV antibody counseling and testing program may read the relevant section to help plan the educational component of the new service.

Others may want to read the guide from beginning to end. A striking finding from the interviews conducted for this guide was that many AIDS educators have difficulty planning and evaluating programs and responding to political pressures. The guide as a whole will give readers the opportunity to consider their work more reflectively and analytically and to develop comprehensive prevention programs rather than simplistic one-shot interventions.

Many helped to make this guide a reality. The American Public Health Association (APHA) Executive Board provided me with a small grant to support the initial interviews. The APHA Program Development and Publications Boards offered useful criticism on several chapters of the guide; Cecil Sheps, Kristine Gebbie, Bruce Chin, and Al Ockerse in particular made useful suggestions for its improvement. Walter Lear helped design this project and has provided useful guidance throughout. Jackie Alexander, Director of Publications at APHA, was a thoughtful and helpful editor.

The Hunter College School of Health Sciences made significant contributions of space, release time, and material support for this project, including a sabbatical that allowed me to complete it.

Several of my students played an important role in gathering data, conducting interviews, and reading sections of the manuscript. They are Felicia Berger, James Holmes, Carol Ambrose, Claire Jagemann, Liliane Kodner-Droyen, Lisa Moore, Robert Lederer, and Beth LaPlaca. Jacalyn Lee and Liz Schnee, my research associates, were involved in every stage of the preparation of this guide. They interviewed AIDS educators, reviewed relevant literature, and helped prepare case histories and tables. Without their ongoing assistance, this guide would not exist. Shavon Glover, Cheryl Key, Sheryl Heron, and Robert Lederer helped ready the manuscript.

A few people have been particularly helpful in defining my views on AIDS and AIDS education over the past six years. They are Wendy Chavkin, Jim Monroe, Rebecca Reiss, Beth Richie, Jacalyn Lee, Liz Schnee, Naomi Lichtenstein, Michael Carrera, Rafael Tavares, Cindy Patton, Archie Harrison, and the leaders and staff of Gay Men's Health Crisis. Our discussions have forced me to expand my thinking about health education, AIDS, and AIDS control.

Because the guide is based on interviews with interested parties to a variety of controversial issues, there will inevitably be different interpretations of the events described and lessons learned. I apologize in advance for any inadvertent misrepresentations. Any errors in judgment are my own.

The prevention of HIV infection is an ongoing task. Readers are urged to send their reactions to, criticisms of, and experiences using this guide to me at Box 609, Hunter College, 425 East 25th St., New York, NY 10010. Their comments will provide a starting point for a guide to the challenges of preventing AIDS in the next decade.

Nicholas Freudenberg

People and Organizations Interviewed

The following individuals were interviewed in person or by telephone or responded to a written survey. In addition, some organizations sent program materials. The organizations listed represent an individual's affiliation at the time of the interview. In the text, sources for quotations are also identified by their affiliation at the time interviewed. Many respondents have since moved to other organizations.

ALABAMA

Montgomery

- Alabama Department of Public Health

ARKANSAS

Little Rock

- Arkansas Department of Health

ARIZONA

Phoenix

- Arizona Department of Health

CALIFORNIA

Berkeley

- Labor Occupational Health Program (AIDS Labor Education Project)
  Elaine Askari

Garden Grove

- AIDS Response Program

Los Angeles

- Aid for AIDS Program
  Bill Green
- AIDS Project Los Angeles
  Daniel Lotta
  Jim Pickett
  Bob Schoonhover
  Judy Spiegel
- Gay and Lesbian Community Services
  Jeff Campbell
- Hemophilia Department/Orthopaedic Hospital
- Los Angeles Department of Health
  David Christy
  Richard Goldberg
  Zayzay Gosa
  Susannah Mejia
- Minority AIDS Project
  Rev. Carl Bean
- Student Health Education Program (SHEP)

Oakland

- AIDS Project of the East Bay
  John Petersen
- Body Electric
  Joe Kramer

San Diego

- San Diego County Health Department

San Francisco

- AIDS Curriculum Project
  Cheri Pies
- AIDS Health Project
  Judy Macks
- Association of Women's AIDS Research and Education/Sex Industry Study (Project AWARE and SIS)
  Laurie Hauer
  Lauren Poole
- Bay View Hunter's Point Multicultural AIDS Prevention Project
  Henri Norris
- Black Coalition on AIDS
  Amanda Houston-Hamilton
- COYOTE/California Prostitute Education Project
  Priscilla Alexander
- Forensic AIDS Project
  Ralle Greenberg
  Bridget Wagner
- Haight Ashbury Clinic
  John Newmeyer
- Levi-Strauss and Company
  Roberta Rich-Johnson
- National Gay Rights Advocates
- San Francisco AIDS Project
  Ruth Schwartz
  Nancy Shaw
- San Francisco Department of Health
  Michael Bala
- Shanti Project
  Andrew Pelfini
- STOP AIDS Project
  Bert Bloom
- Women's AIDS Network
  Nancy Shaw

Santa Ana

- AIDS Project

Santa Barbara

- Tri-County AIDS Project

CONNECTICUT

Hartford

- Connecticut State Department of Health

New Haven

- AIDS Project of New Haven
  George Appleby

DELAWARE

Wilmington

- Delaware Lesbian and Gay Health Advocates
- Delaware State Department of Health

FLORIDA

Miami

- Health Crisis Network
  Page Cole
  Sally Dodds
  Marilyn Volker
- Up Front Drug Information

GEORGIA

Atlanta

- AIDS Atlanta
  Phil Kaufman

HAWAII

Honolulu

- Life Foundation

IOWA

Des Moines

- Central Iowa AIDS Project
  Paula Kelly

ILLINOIS

Chicago

- American Hospital Association
  Linda Brooks—Director, Infection Control

INDIANA

Indianapolis

- Bag Ladies, Inc.

KANSAS

Topeka

- Kansas State Department of Health

KENTUCKY

Frankfort

- Kentucky Department of Health Services

LOUISIANA

New Orleans

- NO/AIDS Task Force
  Aaron Portier
  Larry Pate

MAINE

Portland

- AIDS Project

MARYLAND

Baltimore

- Health Education Resource Organization (HERO)
  Bernard Branson
  Bobbi Klihis
  Christina Rozsenich
  James Shellington
  Jack Stein
  Dace Stone
  Arthur Stutsman

Rockville

- American College Health Association

MASSACHUSETTS

Boston

- AIDS Action Committee
  Bryanne Carmella
  Jeff Epperly
  Dennis James
  Anne Marie Silvia
- Cindy Patton, Author, *Sex, Drugs and AIDS*
- Massachusetts State Department of Health
  Stephen Wroblewski
- Boston Department of Health and Hospitals
  Linette Liebling

MICHIGAN

Ann Arbor

- University of Michigan School of Public Health
  Noreen Clark

Royal Oaks

- Wellness Networks

MINNESOTA

Minneapolis

- Minnesota AIDS Project

MISSISSIPPI

Jackson

- Mississippi Gay Alliance
  Eddie Sandifer
- State Department of Health

NEW HAMPSHIRE

Concord

- New Hampshire State Department of Health

NEW JERSEY

East Orange

- New Jersey State Department of Health/Community Health Education Project
  Bob Baxter
  Kristy Lowe

New Brunswick

- Hyacinth Foundation
  Melanie Patajon

Trenton

- AIDS Education Program
  Katherine McCabe

NEW MEXICO

Albuquerque

- New Mexico AIDS Services
  Larry Pock

NEW YORK

Cortlandt

- Cortlandt County AIDS Task Force
  Beverly Overbo
- Mid-Hudson Valley AIDS Task Force

Huntington

- Long Island Association for AIDS Care
  Jonathan Silin

Mineola

- Nassau County Department of Health
  Sandra Gagliardo

New York City

- AIDS Resource Center
- AIDS Service Delivery Consortium
  Kathe Karlson
- American Red Cross of Greater New York Association for Drug Abuse Prevention & Treatment (ADAPT)
  Yolanda Serrano
  Edith Springer

- Bellevue Hospital
  - Gretchen Harris
  - Jeanne Kalinoski
- Beth Israel Medical Center
  - Errol Chin Loy
- Brooklyn AIDS Task Force
  - Yannick Durant
  - Ernesto de la Vega
- Community Health Project
  - Denise Ribble
- Covenant House
  - Joan Altman
- District Council 37 AFSME
  - Judy Malkin, Program Coordinator
  - Health and Safety Unit
- Emergency Medical Academy (Emergency Medical Technicians)
  - Edward Gabriel
- Local 1199 of Health and Hospitals Workers Union
  - Laura Job
- Gay Men's Health Crisis
  - Richard Dunne
  - Jim Holmes
  - Raymond Jacobs
  - Chuck McKinney
- Haitian Women's Program, American Friends Service Committee
  - Patricia Benoit
  - David Harris
  - France Peon
- Hispanic AIDS Forum
  - Ruth Rodriguez
  - Rafael Tavares
- Hunter College School of Health Sciences
  - Michael Carrera
- Minority AIDS Task Force
  - Suki Ports
- Montefiore Medical Center/Residency Program in Social Medicine
  - Susan Pincus
- National Council of Churches
- National Hemophilia Foundation
  - Christopher Whitney
- New York City Board of Education
  - Geri Abelson
- New York City Department of Health
  - Karen Denard
  - Chris Jacques
  - Sunny Rumsey
  - Bruce Shutte
- New York State Department of Substance Abuse Service
  - Samuel Friedman
  - Douglas Goldsmith
- New York University
  - Stephanie Miller
- Sanitation Workers
  - Joseph Timpone
- West Side AIDS Project
  - Judy Wenning
- Women's Action Alliance
  - Gerry Pearlberg
- Women's AIDS Project
  - Marilyn Auerbach
  - Claire Jagemann
- Young Adult Institute
  - Perry Samowitz

Stony Brook

- AIDS Education Project/State University of New York
  - Bette Coppola
- AIDS Education Resource Project/SUNY
  - Barbara Mautner
- State University of New York at Stony Brook
  - Rose Walton

Syracuse

- AIDS Task Force of Central New York

NORTH CAROLINA

Charlotte

- Metrolina AIDS Project
  - Leslie Kooyman

Durham

- Lesbian and Gay Health Project

Raleigh

- North Carolina State Health Department
  - David Jolly

OHIO

Akron

- Akron City Department of Health

Canton

- Canton City Department of Health

Cincinnati

- AIDS Task Force/University of Cincinnati
- Cincinnati Health Department

Cleveland

- Cleveland Department of Health
  - Joan Mallick
- Gay and Lesbian Community Service Center
  - Emmett Vicaro
- GEAR/Gay Educational and Awareness Resources Foundation

Columbus
- Ohio State Department of Health

Medford
- People for People With AIDS
  Chris Maquerra

OREGON
Portland
- Cascade AIDS Project
  David Diehnel
  Scott Ekblad

PENNSYLVANIA
Harrisburg
- South Central AIDS Assistance Network (SCAAN)
  Roger Beatty

Philadelphia
- Blacks Educating Blacks About Sexual Health Issues (BEBASHI)
  Rashidah Hassan
- Philadelphia AIDS Task Force
  Nicholas Ifft
  Theodore Johnson
  Walter Lear
- Philadelphia Department of Health
  Penelope Barchfeld-Venet
  Donald Cohen
  Robert Sharrar

Pittsburgh
- Health Education Center
  Jan Buzza
- Pittsburgh AIDS Task Force
  Mark Friedman
- Pittsburgh Men's Study
  Anthony Silvestre

RHODE ISLAND
Providence
- Rhode Island Department of Health

TENNESSEE
Memphis
- Aid to End AIDS Committee

Nashville
- Nashville CARES
  Tommy Powell

TEXAS
Dallas
- Dallas County Health Department
  Marc Lerro
  JoAnn Valentine

Houston
- AIDS Foundation

UTAH
Salt Lake City
- People Concerned About AIDS
  Graham Bell
- Utah Department of Health
  Jessalyn Pittman

VIRGINIA
Norfolk
- Tidewater AIDS Crisis Task Force

WASHINGTON
Seattle
- Northwest AIDS Foundation
- Seattle/King County Health Department AIDS Project
  Ann Downer
- Shanti/Seattle
  Nancy Geller

WASHINGTON, DC
- AFSME
  James August
- Center for Population Options
  Debra Haffner
- National AIDS Network
  Paul Kawata
- National Jewish AIDS Project
- Service Employees' International Union (SEIU)
  Shawn Knox
- Whitman-Walker Clinic

WEST VIRGINIA
South Charleston
- South Charleston State Department of Health
  Dave Brangan

WISCONSIN

Madison

- State of Wisconsin Council on Lesbian and Gay Issues

Milwaukee

- National Coalition of Gay STD Services (NCGSTDS)

WYOMING

Cheyenne

- State Department of Health
  Donna Trout
- Wyoming State Department of Health

S E C T I O N   O N E

Planning AIDS Education Programs

Planning effective AIDS prevention programs requires two very different kinds of skills. First, educators need to understand the social and political forces that shape the environment in which they practice. Often AIDS educators feel they are walking through a minefield: The words they choose to describe risk behaviors, the images on the pamphlets they distribute, the population they decide to target or avoid—any of these decisions can lead to an explosion that can threaten their ability to communicate effectively or even to keep their job. Learning how to respond to these broader forces and to build ongoing political support for their programs is a crucial determinant of an educator's effectiveness.

Second, AIDS educators need to know how to choose objectives, select appropriate education activities, implement programs, and evaluate outcomes—the pedagogical skills that make the difference between success and failure. This section presents an analysis of the experience of AIDS educators during the last eight years as they attempted to combine these two perspectives to plan programs that addressed the multiple factors that influence the behaviors that put people at risk of HIV infection.

C H A P T E R   O N E

The Social and Political Context of AIDS Education

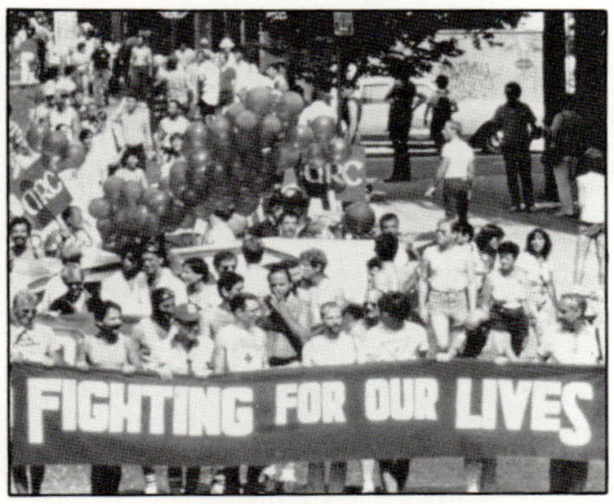

AIDS is too important to be treated as a political problem.

—An AIDS educator

People sometimes decline to contribute to AIDS advocacy organizations, saying they "can't be associated with politics." They might as well say they can't be associated with AIDS, because politics and AIDS are inextricably linked.

—Gary McDonald, former executive director of AIDS Action Council

It is time to put self-defeating attitudes aside and recognize that we are fighting a disease, not people.

—Surgeon General C. Everett Koop, MD, ScD

AIDS is nature's retribution on homosexuals.

—Patrick Buchanan, former White House aide

Some education is going to have to reach the level of pornography or you are going to be missing enormous numbers of people who are at risk.

—Jim Mitchell, producer of safe sex adult films

Any federal educational campaign on AIDS must stress "responsible sexual behavior" based on fidelity, commitment and maturity, placing sexuality within the context of marriage and "should teach that children should not engage in sex."

—Attorney General Edwin Meese, in memo to President Reagan

I would hope that Reagan, as part of his emphasis on family values, would use the AIDS crisis to take the sexual revolution head on because AIDS provides the ideal opportunity to reestablish forgotten verities of moral behavior.

—Gary Bauer, President Reagan's domestic policy adviser

People ask me, "Well, aren't you going against the church by encouraging people to use condoms?" My response is, "I'm concerned about stopping the spread of HIV infection, that's all. If the church is against condoms for contraception, I will not argue with them on that."

—a Latino physician

For the first time in the history of human plagues, science has given policymakers an opportunity to respond without panic and without resort to extreme measures. Not that policymakers are taking advantage of this opportunity for rational action—only that they could if available knowledge were deployed wisely.

—June Osborn, MD, Dean, University of Michigan School of Public Health

By their opposition to open discussion of the issue, religious groups and government have contributed to the AIDS epidemic. AIDS educators have to be willing to challenge these negative attitudes.

—Michael Carrera, sex educator

It would be counterproductive from a public health point of view to see AIDS as a disease of any racial or ethnic group. It's a color-blind message we want to get across. Anybody who engages in risky behavior is at risk.

—Stephen Joseph, MD, MPH, Commissioner of Health, New York City

We don't believe in generic education. People aren't neuter. People in the Black community must recognize AIDS is not a white disease and Black community organizations are most capable of getting that message across.

—Rashidah Hassan, Executive Director, Blacks Educating Blacks about Sexual Health Issues, Philadelphia

First, the experts told us it was safe to watch the atomic bomb explosion. Then they told us Agent Orange posed no danger and that the toxic chemicals at Love Canal were harmless. Now they tell us having AIDS victims use a clinic in our neighborhood presents no risk. How long will it take us to learn?

—New York City council member, at public meeting opposing an ambulatory facility for AIDS patients

Just as the human immunodeficiency virus (HIV) disrupts normal functioning throughout the body, so has the epidemic of acquired immunodeficiency syndrome (AIDS) challenged this country's social and political systems. Although no disease exists in a vacuum, for a variety of reasons our society's response to AIDS is particularly deeply embedded in our social foundations. For one reason, the primary groups affected by AIDS in this country have been drug users and gay men, each stigmatized by the dominant society. For another, the syndrome has been linked to sexual behavior and illicit drug use, both highly charged subjects. Like a magnifying glass, the AIDS epidemic has magnified other social problems—the lack of an equitable and rationally financed health care system, the lack of consensus on broad-based sex education, the tendency to blame social problems on their victims, a housing crisis, and the public distrust of scientists and other experts.

As the opening quotes illustrate, AIDS and politics are "inextricably linked." Broad social and political forces have shaped the epidemic's spread and determined our society's responses to AIDS. This chapter illustrates how these larger issues influence both the day-to-day work of AIDS educators and the environment in which this work is carried out. It then examines how educators have reacted to these external forces and suggests how they can function effectively in a political climate.

Homosexuality

Perhaps the most visible determinant of our society's initial response to AIDS was homophobia, the irrational fear and hatred of lesbians and gay men. By the early 1980s, the gay rights movement had won many important victories. Openly gay communities had become established in big cities throughout the country. In some cities, gay-identified candidates had been elected to political offices and legislation banning discrimination against lesbians and gay men had been passed.

But these successes provoked a backlash. New Right leaders like Anita Bryant, Jerry Falwell, Patrick Buchanan, and Phyllis Schlafly bitterly attacked the new freedoms won by gay people. In 1977, Miami passed a referendum denying equal rights to gay men and lesbians and only a determined effort by progressive political groups in California prevented passage of a 1978 proposition that would have banned homosexuals or those who "encouraged" homosexuality from teaching in public schools. In New York City, a bill barring discrimination against gay people was introduced each year, and every year opposition from religious and conservative groups blocked its passage.

It was in this climate of struggle and backlash that what was soon labeled "gay-related immune deficiency" was first reported in 1981. Doctors diagnosed this new condition, marked by repeated opportunistic infections or a previously rare cancer (Kaposi's sarcoma), in gay men in New York, Los Angeles, and San Francisco. Both physicians and the media quickly tapped into prevalent currents of homophobia. Medical staff in some of New York City's teaching hospitals dubbed the syndrome "wog disease," standing for "wrath of God," and several newspapers and magazines ran stories on "the gay plague."

The Reagan Administration's slow response to AIDS was determined by several political factors, but certainly its antipathy to homosexuality contributed to its unwillingness to promptly appropriate significant resources for the control of a disease that seemed to be limited to a politically unpopular population. As Congressman Henry Waxman observed in 1982, "There is no doubt in my mind that if the same disease had appeared among Americans of Norwegian descent, or among tennis players, rather than among gay males, the response of . . . the government . . . would have been different." Only when the potential for the epidemic to spread outside the "risk groups" became clear and when congressional criticism increased did the Reagan Administration begin to devote new resources to AIDS research and control.

Throughout the epidemic, homophobia has both shaped and been shaped by the social response to AIDS. In 1986, the US Supreme Court upheld Georgia's sodomy law, which makes homosexual acts between consenting adults a felony. Reported complaints of discrimination against and physical assaults on lesbians and gay men increased throughout the 1980s, and national public opinion polls also indicated increased fears of gay people. For example, in a 1985 *Newsweek* poll, 13% of the respondents reported that the fear of AIDS had led them to avoid people they perceived to be gay, and 28% avoided places where gay people might be present.

Government indifference and social ostracism forced the gay community itself to begin the mobilization against AIDS. The Gay Men's Health Crisis (GMHC) was founded in New York City in 1981, the San Francisco AIDS Foundation and Los Angeles CARES soon after. These organizations and others like them created the first education materials on AIDS, provided the first support services for people with AIDS, and lobbied for increased government funding for research and services.

But this vital mobilization of the gay community contributed to the public perception that AIDS was a problem only of homosexuals. Mass media coverage of AIDS reinforced this belief and helped spread it throughout the nation. The homophobic undercurrents of this coverage were revealed by frequent references to "innocent victims" of AIDS such as infants and hemophiliacs, as opposed to the gay men who, by implication, had nothing to blame for their conditions but their own behavior.

This notion that AIDS was a gay disease has profoundly influenced the work of AIDS educators. As gay writer Dennis Altman pointed out: "The central dilemma in thinking about AIDS is that while it is medical nonsense to think of it as a 'gay disease,' it is the gay experience of AIDS, rather than, say, that of drug users, hemophiliacs or Zairians, that has shaped the perceptions and the politics of the epidemic."

Even as late as 1989, for most Americans, the first association with the word AIDS is homosexuality; indeed, men who have sex with other men still represent nearly 70% of people with AIDS in the US. Before educators can hope to convey new information, much less change behaviors, they must help learners work through the complex set of feelings that homosexuality evokes. Before heterosexuals—white, African-American, or Latino—are willing to listen to AIDS messages, they must be able to let go of the myth that AIDS is a disease only of gay men.

Before our society as a whole, and its government in particular, are willing to find the resources needed to control AIDS, they must reject the belief that gay men are an expendable part of our population. Although only certain elements of the New Right have actually articulated this view, homophobia exists throughout the population. A 1985 national public opinion survey by the *Los Angeles Times* found that 28% of the respondents agreed either strongly or somewhat with the statement that "AIDS is a punishment God has given homosexuals for the way they live."

The AIDS epidemic has forced our society to confront the issue of homosexuality as never before. As a result, there is now more open discussion of sexual behavior and values, and more explicit descriptions of gay sexuality than ever possible earlier. On the other hand, AIDS has provided yet another reason—the perception of probable death—for proselytizing against homosexuality.

How AIDS educators respond to this new public awareness about homosexuality will determine both their ability to communicate effectively and the social climate in which lesbians and gay men will live for the coming decades.

Race

From its earliest days, race and racism have been central forces shaping American society. Every aspect of our history has been touched by the economic inequality that African-Americans and other people of color are subject to and by the prejudice and discrimination they encounter. Thus, it is hardly surprising that race and racism have played a key role in shaping the social response to AIDS.

Nationwide, by the end of 1988, the Centers for Disease Control reported that 40% of all persons diagnosed with AIDS, 70% of women with AIDS, and 75% of children under age 13 with AIDS were African-American or Latino. However, African-Americans and Latinos constitute less than 20% of the American population. And whereas 78% of white AIDS patients are reported to be gay or bisexual, fully half of African-American and Latino people with AIDS are heterosexual. These data led one observer to note that "there are two AIDS epidemics in America," one among whites and the other among people of color.

How to respond to this disproportionate impact of AIDS on people of color has provoked sharp conflict among AIDS educators. Some, like New York City Health Commissioner Dr. Stephen Joseph, have argued for a "color-blind" control strategy. The higher rate of AIDS among Blacks and Latinos, they claim, is an artifact of drug use, and it is on this risky behavior, rather than on race, that education should be focused. Proponents of this view believe that calling attention to the racial dimensions of AIDS will further stigmatize both people with AIDS and people of color. They fear that emphasizing the increased risks of African-Americans and Latinos will reinforce the racist view that most people of color use illegal drugs. Moreover, if AIDS is "ghettoized," they argue, the likelihood of winning needed resources will be diminished.

AIDS educators working with African-American and Latino communities frequently report resistance to the notion that AIDS is a problem. A volunteer with a gay AIDS group who sought to meet with the congressional representative from a Black district in 1984 reported that he was "told in no uncertain terms that this problem did not in any way affect his population and he [the congressman] did not have the time to deal with a grassroots gay organization."

Dr. Wayne Greaves, chief of infectious diseases at Howard University Hospital, offered an explanation for this denial. "I think Blacks are afraid to speak out for fear of being identified with the problem," he said, "as if to talk about it means you condone what's happening. Or as if you were betraying yourself to admit that there's a problem in the Black community."

But many African-American and Latino AIDS educators reject both the denial strategy and the "color-blind" argument. Based on their interpretation of the Black experience in America, they believe that the status of people of color improves when racial issues are openly confronted, not when they are ignored. "We have to make AIDS a Black community health issue," said Rashidah Hassan, director of Blacks Educating Blacks About Sexual Health Issues (BEBASHI), a group doing AIDS education in the African-American community in Philadelphia. Otherwise, she warned, "AIDS will be like heart disease, diabetes, cancer and so many other diseases where we have accepted that Black people die at higher rates than whites." And Eleanor Holmes Norton, former chair of the US Equal Opportunity Employment Commission, said, "Only if [AIDS] information is provided by Black organizations" can "Blacks take charge of how their community is educated" and thus avoid "a stigma problem."

Another argument for acknowledging the specific impact of AIDS on people of color is the necessity to develop culturally appropriate education strategies. According to Hassan of BEBASHI, each group knows its own culture, myths, and legends and can thus best plan its own education. "We have to use the culture to present the facts," explained Ruth Rodriguez of New York City's Hispanic AIDS Forum.

The failure to develop such targeted education accounts in part for the difficulty of reaching people of color. In a comment echoed by educators around the country, a New Orleans AIDS activist said, "The one criticism of our brochures is that they only work for white middle class audiences."

Given the limited efforts of both mass media and most AIDS organizations to reach out to people of color, it is not surprising that public opinion surveys show that African-Americans are less well informed about AIDS than whites. According to one national survey in 1985, 65% of African-Americans reported that they knew hardly anything or nothing at all about AIDS compared to 49% of the general population. A statewide survey in Illinois in 1987 also showed that African-Americans, Latinos, people with low incomes, and particularly young people reported that they knew little about AIDS.

To remedy this problem, some African-American and Latino AIDS activists have left primarily white organizations to form new groups that specifically address the needs of their communities. "Everything the Philadelphia AIDS Task Force did reinforced the notion that AIDS was a white gay disease," said Hassan of BEBASHI, "so I felt we needed a new group to work in the Black community." An African-American AIDS worker in New York City who had worked with GMHC decided that "it is easier to teach AIDS to culturally sensitive organizations than to teach cultural sensitivity to GMHC."

Race influences AIDS education in other ways. The history of racial discrimination has led some to fear that AIDS will lead to further stigmatization of African-Americans, Latinos, and other people of color. For example, mandates for widespread screening of women for HIV antibodies in family planning and prenatal clinics has raised the specter of mostly white health professionals urging mostly African-American and Latino women to postpone childbearing indefinitely or to have abortions. Given the current anti-abortion climate (particularly the difficulty poor women face in getting abortions) and given the history of sterilization abuse against women of color, AIDS educators need to find new ways to talk about the real threat of AIDS without rekindling fears of genocide.

Conflicts about race have split AIDS organizations around the country and have hampered the development of effective education programs. African-Americans and Latinos have felt that they receive inadequate funding for their efforts, that they are represented in decision making only in token ways, or that the special needs of their communities are not taken into account.

In some cases, Black homophobia and white racism have clashed head on. White AIDS educators have felt resentful at having their motivation or commitment challenged. When volunteers from GMHC attempted to conduct outreach in African-American communities, one reported: "We were both physically and verbally abused by the community we were trying so hard to reach. How many times and for how long must you try before you give up trying to help and educate? How much abuse is one expected to endure before going on to other projects that people are willing to learn from?" But the reality is more complex than the question of whether African-American people are "willing to learn" from whites; the educator's unconscious racist attitudes and the historic insensitivity of many white professionals may play at least as much a role in the anger of African-Americans as homophobia.

In the United States today, there is no escape from the issue of race. The response of AIDS educators of all colors to race and racism will determine their ability to educate the multihued people of this country. As subsequent case histories illustrate, several African-American and Latino groups in Detroit, Philadelphia, Los Angeles, and elsewhere have already developed innovative approaches to AIDS education.

Drugs

Had biology and human behavior interacted differently to make AIDS appear first among, say, white middle-class children or men attending an American Legion convention, society's response would have been very different. But it was gay men and IV drug users who first became ill and who continue to constitute the large majority of cases. The American view of drug addicts has decisively shaped the response of AIDS educators to the needs of this group.

Long before HIV infection entered the drug-using population, life for the addict was perilous. Contaminated drugs, overdose, homicide and assault, endocarditis, hepatitis, and other infectious diseases had contributed to high death rates among this group. The very fact of taking drugs made users criminals; in addition, many addicts turned to theft, prostitution, selling drugs, or other illegal activities to support their habit.

For many health care providers, drug addicts are the least desirable patients. They fail to comply with treatment, they abuse their caregivers, they deliberately damage their own health, and they consume vast amounts of health care resources. This dislike for drug users contributed to the decision in the 1970s to set up a separate system outside regular health care for treating drug addicts.

The surest way to prevent the spread of HIV infection through drug use is to stop drug use. Yet in New York City, which has more than 200,000 IV drug users, treatment facilities are available to only 35,000 people. By the end of 1988, no new methadone programs had been opened for nearly a decade. Many drug treatment centers have long waiting lists. Moreover, the success rate of most drug treatment facilities is dismal. More than 40% of those who enter drug treatment drop out of treatment; most studies show that only 20 to 30% remain drug- and crime-free a year later.

In some places, budget cuts by the Reagan Administration have forced states to charge addicts for detoxification services. In New Jersey, for example, detoxification in a methadone program costs $50 to $170, depending on the clinic. In 1980, when it was free, 8,703 New Jersey addicts completed detoxification; in 1984, after the budget cuts, 3,075 did. "An addict has $50," said a state health department worker, "he puts it in his veins."

Because of the lack of treatment facilities, their low success rate, and the unwillingness of many addicts to enter treatment, AIDS educators have proposed teaching addicts the dangers of sharing needles and other equipment, showing them how to clean injection paraphernalia, and even distributing free clean needles. Each of these proposals has encountered strong opposition from law enforcement officials and politicians, who argue that such measures seem to condone illegal drug use.

For a variety of reasons, most addicts have withdrawn from mainstream society to join their own subculture. Characterized by its own jargon, values, norms, and patterns of communication, the drug subculture has been hard to reach with traditional health education methods. These problems have led some public health officials to proclaim that addicts are uneducable, a charge that has made it even harder to mobilize the resources—and the imagination—needed to make progress. Nevertheless, a variety of innovative approaches, including the training of ex-addicts as peer educators and the development of special materials, have been tried with some success. These programs are described more fully in Chapter 6.

Finally, society's larger ills confront practicing and recovering addicts particularly acutely. At a time of high unemployment, shortages of low-cost housing, and lack of health insurance coverage for many of the working poor, the recovered addict who completes treatment will have great difficulty finding a job, a home, and health care. When the potential rewards of quitting drugs are relatively low, the costs of continued exposure to drugs and AIDS may not seem so high.

Health Care

"The link between AIDS and drug abuse and sexual practices has frequently dominated the discussions and obscured the link to past health policy problems," wrote Dr. David McCallum of Georgetown University's Institute for Health Policy Analysis. For example, only in a society with no national system for financing health care could a condition like AIDS threaten to bankrupt hospitals in cities such as Newark, New York, and Los Angeles. The emergence of AIDS at the same time when the Reagan Administration was making substantial cuts in primary and preventive health services weakened the ability of public health officials to respond to the epidemic aggressively and decisively. During the mid-1980s, many state governments faced serious budget crises that hampered their ability to launch programs to meet new needs.

The nation's health care system shapes what health educators can tell people about testing, treatment, and preventive services. It can either facilitate or block the individual and collective changes that are necessary to control the spread of HIV infection.

A few examples illustrate these potentials. In San Franciso, the city health department removed money from sexually transmitted disease (STD) clinics to fund AIDS programs. Yet, as Amanda Houston-Hamilton of San Francisco's Black Coalition on AIDS explained, STD clinics are the main or only source of medical care for many African-American men. "You don't have to wait. Nobody knows your name," and so, she said, "you have a perfect opportunity to do some AIDS education and outreach." The decision to cut STD services was a setback for AIDS prevention. Yet in the early years of the epidemic, much of the federal funding for AIDS was diverted from other important preventive programs.

In many cities, the failure of public health authorities to respond to AIDS led private nonprofit groups to provide counseling, social services, hospice care, and public health education. Indeed, one of the remarkable aspects of AIDS has been the unprecedented mobilization of volunteer efforts to cope with the epidemic. Yet this development raised some troubling questions. Cities like New York and San Francisco have large, affluent, gay communities who can sustain volunteer programs, but will the smaller cities (where AIDS is expected to increase rapidly in the next decade) be able to provide similar services? And what precedent is set when some diseases are seen as a legitimate responsibility of the public health care system but others must be addressed by private initiatives? Is it fair to ask the gay community, through its unpaid volunteer work, to subsidize the social costs of AIDS? Will communities of African-Americans and Latinos be able to launch an equally concerted volunteer effort?

Public policies on HIV antibody screening pose yet another dilemma. In theory, it would make sense for an individual's physician to know the results of any antibody test. This knowledge would allow counseling, advice on risk reduction, and ongoing medical monitoring. Yet few hospitals have any reasonably effective method for protecting the confidentiality of medical records. In many hospitals, a patient is unlikely to see the same medical provider more than once. Even neighborhood health centers and family planning clinics often have difficulty in providing continuity of care. Thus, organizational shortcomings in the health care system have forced the establishment of anonymous test sites, where people can go for testing with reasonable certainty that no one else will find out their results. But the price to be paid for this certainty is the addition of yet another facility to the long list of places most Americans, and especially poor people, must visit to get needed medical care. More important, there is no certainty that those who are tested at anonymous sites will receive the ongoing medical or psychological services they will need.

Sexuality and Reproduction

In Los Angeles, the Catholic Church barred the use of its facilities by an AIDS service organization because the group was distributing condoms at its meetings.

In New York City, the board of education delayed for a year the showing of a highly acclaimed film on AIDS that it had commissioned because of fears that conservative critics might charge that the film did not sufficiently stress the importance of abstinence.

Around the country, AIDS organizations receiving grants from the Centers for Disease Control (CDC) report that they have been impeded in their production of educational materials by requirements that all work be reviewed by a community panel to determine that it does not offend community standards. CDC also bars use of its funds for materials that show pictures of human genitals. Diagrams demonstrating how to roll a condom onto a penis, for example, would be unacceptable. An amendment to an AIDS federal funding bill introduced by Senator Jesse Helms bars federal funding for any activities that are deemed to "promote" IV drug use or homosexual or heterosexual sexual activity.

These and other instances illustrate how AIDS has become a lightning rod for the currents of sexual politics circulating in our society. AIDS educators ignore these currents only at their peril.

On the one hand, AIDS has created new opportunities for sex educators. For the first time, terms like "anal intercourse" and "condoms" are appearing in the mass media. One consequence of AIDS will inevitably be a more straightforward and explicit national vocabulary of sex. As Marian Wright Edelman of the Children's Defense Fund put it, "AIDS may do for us what 1 million teenage pregnancies couldn't do: get us talking about sex. People who were tongue-tied realize they must address something that is lethal."

Long-time sex educators express concern that the AIDS issue may overwhelm some of the positive messages that they seek to communicate. "If sex educators talk only about AIDS, pregnancy, and contraception, they give a very limited view of sexuality," said Michael Carrera, former president of the American Association of Sex Educators and Counselors. "Yet the truth is, if you want to go into schools to say there is joy about using your body to express yourself sexually, people will say, 'Get out of here. We don't want you.' "

Although national public opinion polls have consistently shown that the majority of Americans, including parents, support sex education, the opposition of a determined minority of conservatives has often prevented implementation of such programs. These same groups (including the Moral Majority, the Catholic Church, and fundamentalist religious organizations) have opposed public distribution and television advertising of condoms. As a result, AIDS educators have often had to devote considerable time to overcoming such obstacles to communication on sexuality.

Sexual politics has also influenced how AIDS educators have addressed male and female sex roles. Despite the lack of evidence that female prostitution has played a significant role in the spread of AIDS in the United States, and despite the fact that women constitute less than 10% of the AIDS cases in this country, researchers and public officials seem determined to find a contagious role for female prostitutes. The many AIDS education and outreach programs targeted at prostitutes focus on female prostitutes, although the evidence suggests that male prostitution may be a more important source of infection. Few provide drug treatment services for addicted prostitutes, although drug use plays a critical role in infecting prostitutes.

Safer-sex guidelines also sometimes implicitly endorse stereotyped notions of male and female sexuality. Males, straight and gay, are urged to use condoms so that they can enjoy sex without fear of catching or spreading illness. Women, however, are urged to protect themselves so that their babies will not become infected with the HIV virus. According to Dr. Wendy Chavkin, former director of the Bureau of Maternity Services and Family Planning at the New York City Department of Health, "The unwillingness of AIDS educators to discuss the contraceptive benefits of condoms suggests that it is still too controversial to acknowledge that women too engage in nonprocreational sex."

Some observers have noted that the AIDS epidemic has created the necessity for women to play a more assertive role in sexual relationships. In response to the question "How do you negotiate safe sex with your partner?" Elissa Florez, an actress in pornographic films and a safe-sex educator, said "Negotiate, bullshit. If you take off your panties, you take out a condom."

But as Amanda Houston-Hamilton of the San Francisco Black Coalition on AIDS said, such advice is not always realistic. "For women who have been socialized to think of themselves as victims, having the relationship may be more important than keeping safe. If she's so scared that if she says something about sex he's going to walk out on her and the two babies, then she's not going to say a damn thing."

Once again the power relationships that divide men and women, African-Americans and whites, heterosexuals and homosexuals, shape the climate in which people can receive and act on the messages that AIDS educators broadcast. As will be emphasized throughout this guide, only if educators understand and address these dynamics will their efforts have a chance to succeed.

Scientific Issues

In fall 1985 in Canton, Ohio, New York City, and other cities across the country, parents organized to prevent children with AIDS from attending public schools. Despite assurances from researchers and physicians, they feared that their children might contract AIDS in the school. More than three years later, these protests are still occurring.

In 1984, after media coverage of the role of blood transfusions in the spread of HIV infection, blood donations dropped precipitously. Scientific assurances that donating blood (rather than receiving blood) posed no risk were apparently not accepted by many potential donors. As late as 1987, 65% of the respondents to an Illinois survey believed they could get AIDS from donating blood.

These incidents confirm that deep fears shape the social response to AIDS. But they also indicate that the public's perception of scientists in general and AIDS researchers in particular strongly influence how health education messages are received.

Several factors account for the credibility problems that AIDS researchers and public health officials face. First, many Americans lack deep understanding of science and the scientific process. A 1979 survey by the National Science Foundation found that only 7% of American adults were "scientifically literate." Inadequate science education in the schools and erratic coverage in the mass media make it difficult for most people to understand any new scientific issue. The complexity of AIDS—the necessity of understanding at least some principles of such diverse fields as epidemiology, immunology, virology, and pharmacology in order to make sense of obstacles to prevention, treatment, and cure—makes it all the more difficult to understand the syndrome.

But it is too easy to lay all the blame on popular ignorance or the difficulty of the issue. The mass media have played a crucial role in educating the public about AIDS. According to public opinion polls, newspapers and television are the primary source of information on AIDS for most Americans. The eagerness of the media to grasp any sensational angle on AIDS, to broadcast without disclaimer the exaggerated assertions of scientists or public officials, and to present new research findings without appropriate cautions has contributed significantly to popular misconceptions about AIDS.

Scientists and health officials themselves must also share in the responsibility for public distrust. For example, the long struggle to convince public health experts that the toxic chemicals stored in Love Canal presented a health hazard, the assurances by the nuclear power industry that its nuclear power plants were safe, and the willingness of scientists in the pay of the asbestos, pesticides, contraceptive devices, and tobacco industries to testify that their sponsors' products were safe, all helped to sow seeds of distrust of scientists among the public at large. When AIDS researchers report that the HIV virus is almost certainly not contagious except by established routes of transmission, many people don't believe them, citing one example or another in which scientists were perceived to participate in the cover-up of a health problem.

The specific behavior of AIDS researchers and health officials has often reinforced these public doubts. The contentious debate over credit and patent rights to the antibody test among French and American scientists, Secretary of Health and Human Services Margaret Heckler's 1984 claim that an AIDS vaccine was "around the corner," and the government's characterization of Haitians as a risk group (later withdrawn as unjustified) are examples of political interests superseding scientific judgment.

Such apparently self-serving assertions by scientists and public health officials make it more difficult to explain the genuine uncertainties that arise as researchers investigate AIDS. New understanding of the human immune system, new technologies for laboratory studies, and unprecedented funding for research make it inevitable that our knowledge of AIDS will change rapidly. For a public looking for reassurance or clear guides to action, such changes can easily reinforce the view that scientists do not know what they are talking about and are best ignored.

For AIDS educators, the question of how to respond to scientific uncertainty and public distrust of researchers comes up every day. A few examples illustrate the kinds of questions that perplex those who want to convey accurate and understandable information:

- What is the significance of a positive HIV antibody test?
- What evidence is there that a person's knowledge of antibody status will lead to relevant change in behavior?
- How likely is a pregnant woman infected with HIV to pass on the virus to her baby?
- Is there clear evidence that heterosexual vaginal intercourse is a significant mode of AIDS transmission in the United States?
- Given the discovery of more and different strains of viruses related to AIDS, how confident can we be that existing testing programs do in fact protect the blood supply or give individuals relevant information?
- Can kissing in which saliva is exchanged lead to HIV infection?

While scientists and clinicians continue to debate each of these questions, concerned individuals want answers that will help them make major life decisions now. In previous instances of scientific uncertainty, a helpful guideline for public health workers has been to act on incomplete evidence if the potential risks of inaction were high and if the intervention itself seemed to pose acceptable risks. A classic example of this approach is John Snow's removal of the water pump's handle during the epidemic of cholera in London in 1854.

Unfortunately, this rule of thumb does not always help in the current situation. To advise an HIV-antibody-positive woman to defer pregnancy indefinitely (as CDC recommends) might mean saving her from having a baby with AIDS, but it might also mean depriving her forever of the experience of having a healthy child. Encouraging a gay man or a drug user to get the antibody test might lead to reductions in risky behavior, but it might also, for no good public health reason, lead to depression, ostracism, attempted suicide, and discrimination or even increases in risky sexual or drug behavior. How do we weigh these options, and who has the right to decide how to advise people?

These dilemmas suggest that AIDS educators need to take on the additional task of understanding, interpreting, and critiquing the unfolding scientific investigation of AIDS. No longer is it professionally or ethically acceptable for educators to simply act as mouthpieces for scientists and researchers. Indeed, which researcher or point of view would be presented?

Rather, educators must participate in evaluating current research and then make recommendations on messages to be conveyed to the public.

Perhaps even more important, AIDS educators must help their clients to understand the process of science, the nature of uncertainty, and the methods of risk assessment. This is indeed a tall order, but anything less threatens to undermine educators' credibility. The success of the gay community in educating itself about AIDS demonstrates the possibility of conveying massive amounts of information on epidemiology, clinical treatments, safer sex, and the nature of scientific research to a wide audience. Newspapers, community forums, counseling, and word of mouth all contributed to this process. How to replicate such an intensive and sophisticated education effort in communities with lower educational attainments and different learning styles than in educated urban gay areas represents a challenge for AIDS educators in the years to come.

Unless people understand how scientists learn about AIDS, each new piece of information and each change in recommendations will be seen as evidence that public health authorities really do not know what they are talking about. The misperception that donating blood could lead to AIDS and the hysteria provoked by admitting children with AIDS to public schools dramatically illustrate the potential for failure in communication between scientists and the public. Health educators need to take the initiative to prevent such episodes in the future.

The Impact of Politics on AIDS Educators

For AIDS educators, the social and political forces that surround and permeate the epidemic often make their daily work seem like walking through a minefield. At any moment in the course of doing their job, a single action—using sexually explicit language, passing out condoms, teaching a drug user how to clean a needle and works, addressing or not addressing the racial dimensions of AIDS, deciding to provide services to one community rather than another—can set off an explosion that diverts them from their education efforts. Moreover, these larger forces influence health behavior both directly and indirectly. Some of these relationships are illustrated in Figure 1. Failing to acknowledge these social and economic factors can lead to unsuccessful programs. How have educators coped with this anxiety-provoking situation? What strategies have they developed to survive and carry on?

One response to the political pitfalls that entrap educators has been extreme caution. Rather than offend the Catholic Church, CDC, or local elected officials, some organizations have developed materials and programs that will offend no one. The attraction of this choice is that it minimizes the likelihood that time and energy will be diverted from education itself. The problem, however, is that in offending no one, the message is so bland or so vague that no one pays any attention to it. Inoffensive education can easily become ineffective education.

Moreover, by accepting the status quo, educators ensure that some of the most powerful and vocal sectors of society will have veto power over the content and process of education. This is particularly problematic because homogenized education is least likely to have an impact on the stigmatized populations at highest risk of AIDS: gay men and IV drug users. Refusal to discuss sexual behavior explicitly, to teach addicts how to clean their works, or to address the racial dimensions of AIDS makes it unlikely that education will lead to real changes in behavior related to HIV infection.

Figure 1. SOCIAL AND POLITICAL FACTORS THAT INFLUENCE AIDS EDUCATION

Social and Political Factors	Individual Characteristics, Attitudes, or Behaviors	Risks for AIDS
Poverty	■ Inadequate health care and social services ■ Inadequate education ■ Drug abuse ■ Prostitution ■ Incarceration	■ Poor health status ■ Lack of knowledge about health, AIDS, and prevention ■ Not reached by many prevention campaigns ■ Potential to unknowingly infect others ■ Late presentation and diagnosis of AIDS ■ No opportunity for treatment
Racism	■ Distrust of government, health care, and social service system because of historical and current discrimination ■ Internalized oppression leading to low self-esteem ■ Poverty (see above)	■ Belief in genocide theories ■ Mistrust of AIDS information from government ■ Fears about control of reproduction ■ Self-defeating attitudes, negativity, passivity
Homophobia	■ Inadequate and inappropriate health and social services ■ Reluctance to identify as gay or bisexual ■ Community denial of existence of homosexuality ■ Reluctance to seek health care or social services for fear of stigma ■ Physical assaults	■ Information targeted to gay and bisexual men not perceived as relevant ■ Heterosexual activity as cover for homosexuality ■ Community does not acknowledge need for education
Sexism	■ Strict adherence to traditional sex roles including double standard in which men have multiple partners ■ Sexual assault ■ Failure of men to use condoms	■ Women powerless to negotiate in sexual relationships ■ Women at home, thus not available for education ■ Women value motherhood, thus reluctant to defer childbirth
Religion and culture	■ Value placed on children ■ Lack of fluency in English ■ Adherence to strict traditional sex roles ■ Unwillingness to discuss sexuality or drug use	■ Religious prohibitions on birth control and abortion ■ Reluctance to defer childbirth ■ Miss prevention messages because they are mostly in English ■ Denial because of reluctance to confront issues

In a similar, though more subtle, reaction to political opposition, some groups have narrowed their definition of goals. By choosing activities that are less likely to provoke controversy, some AIDS organizations have hoped to create a space to work unfettered by constraints. Government funding that sets limits on explicit language, political activity, or lobbying provides a powerful incentive for these choices. For example, some AIDS organizations have emphasized taking care of people with AIDS, rather than community prevention education, because few opposed these services. Others have avoided working with heterosexuals because of the hostility AIDS educators sometimes encounter from them.

It is not that these are "wrong" choices, especially since there is an almost unlimited need for any AIDS-related service. Rather, by consciously or unconsciously bowing to political pressures, AIDS organizations preclude using a rational planning process in which scarce resources are allocated according to need. And because prevention rarely has a strong constituency, nor does it seem as urgent as meeting the needs of sick people, it is often a casualty in politically expedient decisions.

Recommendations for Surviving in a Political Climate

How then can AIDS educators survive in this political climate? How can they address the larger forces that shape their work without being overwhelmed by them? The following recommendations summarize the experience of AIDS educators and organizations around the country.

Acknowledge the political dimensions of AIDS.

Larry Kramer, a founder of GMHC, has said, "There is nothing in this AIDS mess that is not political." Like it or not, AIDS educators cannot escape the sexual, racial, religious, and partisan politics that shape their environment. Politics will influence our work as surely as the discoveries in research laboratories and hospital wards. If we are concerned about having an impact, to say that we are "above politics" makes as much sense as saying we are "above science."

What concrete steps can AIDS organizations take to recognize the importance of political factors? One important step is to encourage open political discussion in their organizations. By discussing homophobia, racism, and other social problems, AIDS workers can define the real obstacles they face. Denial is a frequent strategy for all groups touched by AIDS, but denying the political aspects of AIDS prevention leaves programs poorly prepared to defend themselves. As one AIDS educator put it, "If you don't take on the politics of AIDS, these politics will sweep you away." Too often, the conflicts between gay and straight, white and nonwhite, male and female staff about priorities and strategies are viewed as unimportant. Moving these discussions out of the hallways and into the boardroom sends a message that the organization is willing to confront these problems.

Teach educators the political skills they need.

Some AIDS educators have a history of political involvement and feel comfortable taking on these tasks. But others lack basic political skills. Some skills that educators need are how to—

- organize networks and coalitions;
- lobby for or against new legislation;
- advocate prevention policies and programs;
- use the media effectively to raise political issues;

- assist groups such as IV drug users to organize for needed services.

Professional groups like APHA and the Society for Public Health Education can play an important role in developing such training programs.

Organize coalitions and networks to advocate for policies and programs that will prevent the spread of HIV infection.

By themselves, AIDS educators and even AIDS organizations have limited power to influence political decisions. But by joining with other groups that share related concerns, the likelihood of political victories is greater. Coalitions and networks need to be organized at the local, state, regional, and national levels. Already some AIDS organizations have taken important steps in this direction.

At the local level, drug abuse treatment programs, youth groups, civil rights and gay rights organizations, health centers, women's groups, and public health professionals are among the potential participants in coalitions for AIDS prevention. Helping community-based organizations that are not AIDS-designated to define a role for themselves in AIDS prevention is a crucial task. To convince these groups to add AIDS prevention to their agenda requires defining the problem in a way that is consistent with each group's mission.

AIDS educators need to find new ways to link our work on AIDS with other related issues such as teenage pregnancy, improved access to contraception, sex education, drug abuse prevention and treatment, and equal rights for women, lesbians, gay men, and people of color. Success in the efforts of the groups working on these issues is essential for the control of AIDS. Each constituency has a cadre of skilled educators, organizers, and activists who can strengthen the work of AIDS prevention.

By joining or helping to organize such coalitions and networks, AIDS educators help build the political muscle needed to create a social climate conducive to prevention. These issues are discussed more fully in Chapter 2.

Target policymakers and political leaders for education.

Behaviors that contribute to the spread of HIV infection include voting against legislation that funds preventive measures, fanning public hysteria, and advocating authoritarian (but often ineffective) programs that drive people at risk away from places where they might be educated and counseled. In order to change these behaviors, AIDS workers need to educate legislators, administrators, and other policy makers.

Some of this education can be direct. Several AIDS organizations have sponsored seminars on AIDS for political leaders. Others send staff to meet with elected representative to explain their position on issues. Some have become sophisticated political operators. One respondent reported that she had learned that "everybody in power, the mayor, the governor, the health commissioner, the hospital administrator, needs to get stroked to reinforce our support." Her organization gets strong financial and political support from the state and local government.

Other education is more indirect. The mass media are a powerful tool for influencing politicians. For too long, health educators have emphasized the role of mass media in providing consumer information or changing attitudes while ignoring the media's agenda-setting potential. The gay rights march in Washington in October 1987 is a good example of a media event that demonstrated the power of gay rights groups, at least in major urban areas.

Develop programs that address the political or social factors enabling or blocking preventive behavior.

If political factors are seen as extraneous to the practice of health education, then addressing them will always be a diversion from the primary responsibility. If, on the other hand, educators assume that it is their job to do whatever is necessary to help people to take action to protect their health, then they can ethically move into the political arena. The question of how to work effectively in the political arena needs to be analyzed in each specific situation, but first they need to agree whether this is a part of their job.

In the case of AIDS, an emphasis on enabling factors would require working to ensure access to drug treatment, making sex education widely available, supporting strict rules on confidentiality of test results, and combating discrimination against gay people, drug users, people of color, and women. Some of these relationships are illustrated in Figure 1.

Create systems to help AIDS educators cope with the political forces that assail them.

The politics permeating the social response to the AIDS epidemic creates not only the external environment in which educators work, but also the internal psychological experience of those involved in that work. Many AIDS educators report frequent distress about their work: anger, frustration, despair, vulnerability.

This distress comes partly from working too hard, sleeping too little, losing too many loved ones, and coping with one's own mortality. But it also comes from being engaged in political battles, often without acknowledgment that this is in fact the situation.

AIDS organizations need to find new ways to help their staffs support each other in these ordeals. Collective efforts to define problems, seek solutions, celebrate victories, and mourn losses are one way. Personal support groups that address the complex interactions among psychological and political factors are another. And more individual approaches such as therapy, vacations, and sabbaticals are also important. These issues are discussed in Chapter 2.

CHAPTER TWO

Building Institutional and Community Support for AIDS Prevention

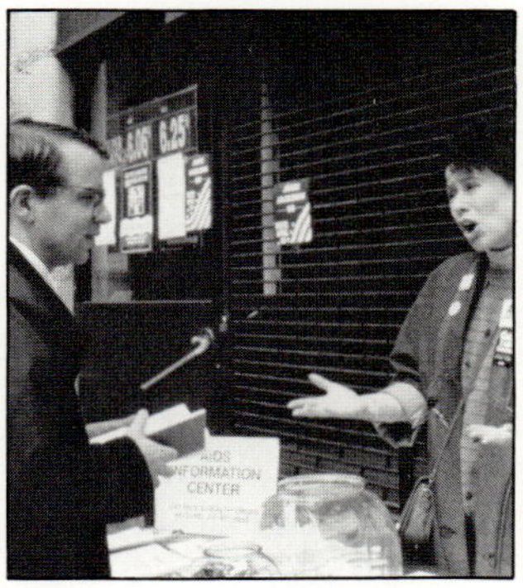

CASE HISTORY

Health Crisis Network, Miami

"For about a year we worked out of the back of a station wagon with only an answering machine to record our messages. In December 1984 we moved into the attic of an old church that has a history of providing safe haven to progressive groups just getting off the ground. That was roughing it. We had no heat or air conditioning—and you know how hot it gets in the summer in Miami. The bathrooms were outside. We were terribly over-crowded and some of our clients had to be carried up the long, steep stairs. We spent nearly two years there, on top of one another. That was a true test of our ability to get along. Sometimes it feels strange in this new building. We're not used to working in separate rooms. Sometimes you'll find us all crowded around this one table. I guess we don't know what to do with all of this space."

This is how Sally Dodds, executive director of the Health Crisis Network (HCN) in Miami, remembered the early days of the organization and the changes the staff have lived through in four years. Today, HCN is Florida's major private AIDS organization.

The rapid transformation from a grassroots group of concerned health workers and gay people to an organization with substantial influence in AIDS care, education, and policy making was, according to Sally Dodds, as much a response to the growing number of people with AIDS in South Florida as to the inadequate public response in the state with the third-highest AIDS caseload in the nation. "Nobody else was doing anything, so we took the initiative ourselves."

Florida had been slow to respond to the epidemic in the southern portion of the state. Between 1981 and 1985, state appropriations for AIDS totaled $576,000. "Florida is a strange place," remarked Dodds. "Seventy-five percent of all the cases of AIDS in the state have been concentrated in and around Miami—a day's car ride from Tallahassee, the state capital. Northern politicians don't understand the South, and Miami paints a unique geopolitical picture. While you might not know it if all you visit is Miami, Florida is in the South."

Dodds attributes HCN's rise to a position of prominence in the midst of a conservative environment to "some good friends in the larger health care system" and the "professional thrust" of HCN's founding members. Her co-workers and clients credit Dodds's skillful community organizing.

Throughout HCN's metamorphosis, its staff has grappled with questions of community and community responsiveness. Like other AIDS organizations, HCN struggles to avoid being identified as only a white gay male organization while 85 to 90% of its volunteers and supporters are from the gay community.

"Some people don't want to refer clients to us because they think we are a gay organization," said Dodds. "Even the CDC tends to define AIDS organizations as gay organizations. They've got to stop doing that. The fact is the gay community has the longest standing expertise with AIDS. For the first time in history, majority society has got to turn to a minority group for the expertise. They don't like doing it. AIDS is forcing us all to look at the diversity of people in our country."

In an effort to serve and adequately represent South Florida's extremely diverse population, HCN has formed a multidenominational clergy advisory committee, asked members from Spanish- and Creole-speaking staff to work in Miami's large Latino and Haitian communities, and formed educational task forces to represent the unique communities of South Florida.

Though quite successful at gaining broad acceptance and support in the medical community, HCN has had less success involving people of color in their work. Dodds noted that "Miami is now 51% Latino. We are a city of immigrants. Racial tensions are high. People are dealing with survival issues. They need jobs, housing, and general health care. We have to confront these realities before we even get to AIDS."

Dodds pointed out that being responsive to one's community and attending to the demands of funding agencies is sometimes difficult. "Public grants can force groups to become institutionalized. We must constantly recognize the fact that we need to seek independent funding sources so that we can preserve our philosophy and value system. Sometimes we may have to choose not to compete for a grant or contract on the basis of its restrictions so we don't have to be in a position to lose responsiveness to our community."

Dodds expressed fears that although it has "never been seen as a radical organization," HCN may be moving toward becoming part of "the establishment."

When people—especially gay people—start coming to us to tell us what the community is thinking, I think, my God, are we becoming so institutionalized that we are "the system"? That's when it's time to get back to the streets. Sure, now that we have this nice, cool office and have made a name for ourselves, it is sometimes tempting to sit back and wait for people to come to us. We all work hard, we're burnt out. But I'll be damned if we let that attitude take over!

Dodds manages her staff of nine paid employees and hundreds of volunteers as if she were leading a small grassroots group. "I spent 15 years working in a hierarchical structure and I know I was never effective then. I'd always be angry at the people above me." Her philosophy at HCN is, "This is your job. You can take as much responsibility as you want. Be creative. Make it what you want it to be. Do what needs to be done. If a problem comes up, let's figure it out. We've never done AIDS work before. We're all making it up as we go along."

Familiarity with health education strategies and detailed understanding of the special needs of the target population are prerequisites for effective AIDS prevention programs. But unless such programs have the support of their institutional sponsors and of the larger community, their goals will be difficult to achieve. The case history describes how one group set about building such support. This chapter discusses some of the problems that AIDS educators have encountered in pursuing this objective and some solutions they have devised. Its objective is to provide educators with practical suggestions for building institutional and community support for AIDS prevention.

In the following discussion, "institutional" problems refer to those issues whose main impact is felt in the agency or group that sponsors the program, and "community" problems define conflicts between an agency and other groups or institutions in the community. Some problems exist at both levels, and both are obviously situated within the larger social and political context described in Chapter 1.

Institutional Problems

Not enough resources for AIDS prevention.

"We don't have enough staff, we don't have enough time, we don't have enough money to do the work we know needs to be done," said an AIDS educator in North Carolina, repeating a complaint heard around the country.

In an institution, lack of resources has the following consequences:

- Needed new programs are not developed.
- Those that are offered are less than adequate. "We are spread too thin to ensure the highest quality," said an AIDS educator in Portland, Oregon.
- Existing staff take on more work than they can realistically manage.
- Significant energy is devoted to fundraising rather than service delivery.
- In multiservice agencies, other services are reduced to expand AIDS-related programs.

Even as significant new government and foundation dollars flow into AIDS prevention, many AIDS organizations still feel chronically starved for the resources they need to do the job right. Obviously, part of the solution is to mobilize politically to convince elected officials to allocate more resources. The success of AIDS organizations and activists in persuading the US Congress to increase funding for AIDS prevention and services for people with AIDS attests to the impact of this strategy.

But at the institutional level, AIDS workers have developed a variety of strategies for coping with inadequate resources. These include—

- using volunteers whenever possible;
- defining more limited objectives;
- sharing resources with other organizations;

- seeking donations of services or supplies;
- choosing low-cost and high-impact education methods—e.g., using peer educators instead of health professionals;
- educating institutional leaders about the importance of allocating more internal resources to AIDS;
- integrating AIDS prevention into existing services, e.g., sex education, health counseling, or prenatal care.

Each of these actions can help groups deliver more services without adding significant new costs. But these cost-cutting measures exact their own burden. Volunteers and peer educators require supervision and training. Limiting objectives means leaving certain tasks undone. Sharing resources with other groups necessitates devoting time and energy to negotiating mutually acceptable relationships.

Too often, AIDS organizations fall prey to one of two fallacies. First, some organizers believe that only additional dollars will allow them to take on more work. The quest for funding becomes all-consuming. This attitude is particularly common in the more professional organizations, where it can unintentionally discourage smaller unfunded groups from taking on *any* effort in AIDS prevention.

Second, others believe that commitment is the sole prerequisite for achieving any task. "In the face of this epidemic, if something needs to be done, we will do it," said one educator. But organizations cannot function on human spirit alone. By failing to mobilize institutional and community support for increased resources, these groups will eventually expend their limited resources.

What's the solution to this dilemma? Unfortunately, it is inherent in the situation: AIDS prevention will never have all the funds it needs, and committed AIDS workers will always want to do more than their resources permit. By balancing human and financial assets against the work that needs to be done, and by choosing a working pace that can be sustained over time, organizations can make the tough choices about what to do today and tomorrow.

Staff burnout, leading to high turnover and low morale.

"Burnout is uppermost in everyone's mind," said an AIDS educator working with hemophiliacs. Working too hard on a controversial and upsetting issue is an obvious cause.

Other causes, perhaps less self-evident, are related to the support that an institution provides (or fails to provide) its staff. "If my staff doesn't feel active or feels alienated," explained Sally Dodds of HCN, "they're not going to get their best work done. That's all there is to it." These are some successful strategies that AIDS organizations have used to prevent burnout:

Ongoing support groups for AIDS workers. In Washington, DC, for example, AIDS educators meet regularly to discuss common problems. The Metropolitan Washington AIDS Educators' Committee sponsors workshops, provides an opportunity for networking, and keeps participants informed of new developments. Such groups help workers to understand that their own problems are not unique and to share methods for reducing or coping with stress.

Liberal vacation and "personal holiday" benefits. Most AIDS workers report that at some point their work becomes unbearable. Being able to take off a few days at that point can contribute to mental rehabilitation just as continuing to work at that time can lead to the decision to quit. Flexible time-off policies make administrators' tasks more difficult in the short run, but they contribute to staff retention and morale in the long run.

Varying staff responsibilities. At the New York Blood Center, HIV counselors share public speaking engagements, research tasks, and attendance at conferences. One counselor said, "If I had to do the same thing every day, I'd go nuts. It's just too depressing. But since we get to do lots of different things, I've been able to stay here for more than two years."

Allowing staff to play a role in setting their own work pace. The occupational health literature demonstrates that control over working conditions helps to reduce stress. By involving AIDS workers in planning their activities, pace, and priorities, managers help to reduce alienation. Managers are also likely to benefit from the staff's own expertise in accomplishing goals efficiently. "It is my philosophy to have staff determine what they need and to tell me, and it's my job to find the resources they need to get the job done," said Dodds of HCN.

Providing staff with adequate supervision, training, and support. "My first six months on the job, I hardly knew anything about AIDS, yet I had to represent my organization at public meetings. It was so humiliating," reported an AIDS educator in Pennsylvania. "I couldn't go to my superior to discuss problems with my clients," said an AIDS counselor in New York, "because I didn't respect her judgment. She had less experience than I did."

Feeling unqualified for one's job, alone without backup, or unappreciated for carrying out an overwhelmingly difficult job can make a worker anxious, angry, and resentful. It can also make him or her want to quit.

By ensuring that staff receive supervision and feedback from a qualified supervisor, training designed to provide the competencies required for the job, and the emotional and professional support needed to maintain morale, agencies can improve staff retention and productivity.

Crisis orientation; no strategic planning or evaluation.

"We're always working from crisis management," reported an AIDS educator in Charlotte, North Carolina. "We don't have time to do evaluations of our programs," an educator in Philadelphia claimed. "I always feel I'm on the end of a tiger," said the director of education for an AIDS group in the South.

These quotes illustrate the pervasive perception of crisis that permeates AIDS organizations. Like staff burnout, it springs in part from having too much to do with too few resources. But although it is based in reality, the crisis mentality has set back the goal of AIDS prevention. It has contributed to poorly planned programs, duplication of services, inability to learn from experience, and a lack of overall direction and priorities. As we approach the end of the first decade of the epidemic, it is imperative that AIDS organizations begin strategic planning.

Among the questions that every organization must consider are the following:

- What populations can our group best serve?
- What services can we offer and what should be left to other groups?
- What group structure will best help us to achieve our goals?
- How can we best learn from our own experiences so as to improve subsequent efforts?
- How can we use our existing resources most efficiently to meet our goals?
- How can we find the resources to carry out our goals for the next five years?
- What do we hope to accomplish in the next five years?

By taking time out from the daily crises that face every AIDS organization, staff can begin to plan in a thoughtful way. These are some activities that have helped groups to plan for the future:

- Hire consultants to advise the group on planning or evaluation. The Baltimore Health Education Resource Organization (HERO), for example, hired a consultant with expertise in organizational development to help it devise a structure for the group that would help it to carry out its goals.

- Organize periodic retreats where staff can discuss long-range problems and goals away from day-to-day job demands.
- Hire full-time staff with expertise in planning or evaluation and specific job responsibilities that include these tasks. Some groups have sent existing staff for professional training in these areas.
- Meet with staff from larger or more experienced groups to seek their advice on planning or evaluation. For example, the National AIDS Network (see "Resources") will assist local groups with relevant expertise. The more established AIDS groups in big cities can also provide this service.

Agency's leadership not sufficiently committed to AIDS prevention as a priority.

Many factors can prevent administrators from wanting to put AIDS prevention high on their agenda: denial that AIDS is a problem in their setting; fear that the agency will be stigmatized by its association with AIDS; unwillingness to offend those who oppose public health (as opposed to moralistic) approaches to prevention; belief that the financial resources for prevention are not available or sufficient; commitments to service delivery, as opposed to prevention, for people with AIDS or other medical problems; or restrictions by funding agencies.

Whatever the cause, AIDS educators working in such settings have the additional job of convincing their administrations to devote more resources to AIDS prevention. A first step in this process is diagnosing the cause of the problem. Distinguishing between informational, political, and financial obstacles will contribute to the development of an effective strategy.

Some administrators may not understand how HIV infection affects their population, the role their agency can play in prevention, or the existing resources that can help to prepare them for this role. In this case, education is appropriate. By giving administrators reports to read, sponsoring seminars for them, and familiarizing them with prevention programs at similar agencies, AIDS educators can equip administrators to play a more active role. Many AIDS trainers now insist on educating management before they begin training staff.

When administrators fear political flak for getting involved in AIDS prevention, the strategy for change must be different. By demonstrating to managers that AIDS prevention programs can also have strong constituencies and bring new financial and public relations benefits to the agency, educators can help to strengthen weak backbones. Some educators have found that AIDS task forces composed of health professionals, elected officials, and community residents can play a useful role in such education.

Similarly, convincing managers that there is also a political price to be paid for *failing* to act on AIDS prevention can raise the political costs of doing nothing. State and federal mandates defining the responsibility of schools, health care providers, and others for AIDS prevention give clout to this argument.

Financial obstacles can also make administrators reluctant to take on AIDS prevention. Family planning centers, for example, are often mandated to provide antibody testing and counseling without the addition of sufficient new resources. The decision to meet this mandate requires reducing other services. Is it surprising that some agencies delay implementing such programs?

AIDS educators can help administrators address this problem by finding external sources of funding for AIDS prevention programs, researching low-cost models for prevention appropriate to their agency, seeking low- or no-cost external human resources (e.g., trainers or consultants) to help implement a program, and searching for ways to integrate AIDS prevention into existing services.

Sometimes administrators feel that a decision to add AIDS prevention to their agency's work requires an immediate commitment to expensive programs: antibody counseling and testing, medical services, extensive staff training, and so on. For some agencies, such an array of services may be desirable, but not feasible in the short run. For others, a less intensive intervention may suffice.

By helping administrators consider a continuum of AIDS prevention activities ranging from low to high cost, educators can ensure that every agency finds something to do. Figure 2 illustrates a list of such activities. Beginning with a few simple activities can help an agency to gain the experience and commitment needed for larger programs.

Figure 2. CONTINUUM OF AIDS PREVENTION ACTIVITIES FOR HEALTH, SOCIAL SERVICE, AND COMMUNITY AGENCIES

LOWER COST

Distribute education materials.
Display posters in agency.
Invite guest speakers to discuss AIDS prevention with staff or clients.
Sponsor community forums on AIDS prevention.
Establish agencywide task force on AIDS.
Establish liaisons with appropriate referral agencies.
Train staff on AIDS prevention.
Join local AIDS network or coalition.
Distribute condoms to clients.
Distribute bleach to IV drug users to allow them to clean works.
Send speakers to local schools or community groups.
Hire AIDS prevention coordinator.
Establish AIDS education and counseling program for agency or community.

HIGHER COST

Organizational action crippled by disagreement about prevention priorities.

Should we expand our program in the gay community, or should we start a new one in the Latino neighborhood?

We need more buddies to take care of people with AIDS, but if we use our ten new volunteers for this, we won't have anyone to send into the schools.

If we want to reach adults, we need to go through the churches, but if we want to reach street kids, they won't talk to us if they think we're part of the church.

Even though we hired a Black outreach worker, we're still not reaching the Black population. Maybe that community isn't ready for AIDS prevention.

Our women's committee has been meeting for a year and still the organization has refused to provide any special services for women. Maybe we should quit and set up our own group.

Dilemmas such as these face AIDS organizations and educators around the country. How they are discussed and decided has a major impact on program effectiveness, staff morale, and the public perception of the organization. The failure to address these issues successfully is probably a major cause of the breakup of AIDS organizations. AIDS educators in New York, Los Angeles, San Francisco, Miami, Philadelphia, and Boston reported spending vast amounts of time and energy on these questions.

Effective resolution requires careful attention to both the content and process of decision making. A clear definition of organizational goals and objectives and a detailed assessment of the target population's needs provide a more objective framework for making decisions on whom to work with and how to work with them. If members of a group disagree about objectives, then it would probably make sense to clarify this issue before making a specific decision on how to allocate resources. If no consensus can be reached, then a group must consider disbanding or perhaps establishing separate committees, each with some portion of the total resources.

A few techniques for more democratic decision making may help to alleviate some of the bad feelings that accompany choosing between alternatives that have strong supporters and opponents:

Give all parties the opportunity to voice their opinion. It's one thing to lose an organizational battle; it's another to feel your viewpoint was not even considered.

Acknowledge the political dimensions of the decision. Homophobia, racism, and sexism are pervasive forces in this society. Deciding to work with one group rather than another will inevitably be linked to these larger currents. When it is made clear that deep-rooted problems are being discussed, these conflicts are depersonalized, allowing perhaps a more rational political discussion. At the same time, the expectation that one organization alone can solve this problem is diminished.

Support political debate as a constructive way to clarify options and contribute to making the best decision. Given the political dimensions of AIDS, no decisions can be made without considering politics. Ignoring these political forces can lead to bad decisions and bad feelings. On the other hand, at some point a group must end debate and make a decision. Some groups have found it helpful to set a time limit on these discussions.

Establish mechanisms for reassessing organizational decisions periodically. The changing patterns of HIV infection, new understanding of the disease, and new resources for prevention all necessitate frequent review of goals and objectives. For example, a group might decide to devote most of its efforts to working with gay men this year, but reevaluate the decision one year from now. When advocates of a losing position know they will have another chance to make their case, they may be less likely to feel angry or resentful or to undermine the course of action that was decided on.

Look for other groups that can take on tasks that your organization cannot handle and look for ways to support these other groups. The value of sharing tasks will be discussed more fully in the section on building community support for prevention, but such a strategy has internal institutional consequences as well. An AIDS organization may decide not to work with a certain population but instead to assist other groups who do. Blacks Educating Blacks About Sexual Health Issues, a group working with African-Americans in Philadelphia, for example, decided to work primarily in the Black community and not in Latino areas. But it trained several Latino leaders in AIDS prevention so that they could work in their community. Such a decision shows staff who support a certain course of action that their concerns are seen as important and will be addressed, even if their agency cannot do it.

Each agency has its own procedures for making decisions, some more democratic and others more hierarchical. But whatever the method, the foregoing strategies can help decision makers involve their staff in considering the issues. No method can eliminate conflict, but by devising mechanisms to enlist all sides in the ongoing process of allocating resources to fight the epidemic, agencies can minimize the costs of dissension.

Agency becoming bureaucratic and losing its human side as it expands.

When the first AIDS organizations were founded in the early 1980s, their staffs were all volunteers, their funds were donated by concerned individuals or raised in the community, and their fuel was commitment and passion. Now many of these groups have multimillion dollar budgets, staffs of several dozen persons, and organizational charts that a corporate efficiency expert would envy. The case history of HCN In Miami illustrates one such group.

Obviously, these changes mean that groups can offer more services, educate more people, and carry out their work more professionally. But growth has a price, too. Among the complaints that staff voice are—

- less attention to advocacy as the group becomes more established, more involvement in service delivery, and more dependence on government funding;
- traditional professional matters such as money, prestige, and turf of more concern to professional staff than before;
- reduced ability to respond quickly or innovatively to emerging needs;
- less personal interaction among staff and managers and therefore less shared decision making;
- more hierarchical structures leading to staff feeling less in control of their work.

As a result of these changes, many AIDS workers experience the success that enables expansion as a negative process, leading to alienation, diminished power, and a loss of idealism.

How can AIDS organizations change this perception? How can they grow without entirely losing their earlier strengths? These are some strategies they have tried:

Delegate some decision-making powers to smaller units of the organization. Many AIDS organizations have set up task forces or committees on African-Americans, Latinos, women, or youth. By allowing these groups to operate somewhat autonomously, the organizations involve more people in decision making, programs are more likely to reflect the needs of those served, and staff in these units are more likely to feel ownership of the program. Assigning these subgroups a budget that they can allocate gives them some real control over institutional resources. This strategy can, of course, lead to its own problems in which the smaller groups become increasingly alienated from the larger organization.

Develop institutional mechanisms that help to maintain close contact among all levels of the organization. Fighting bureaucracy by setting up additional committees may seem contradictory. But cross-sectional groups that advise management on long-range planning, budget, training, and personnel policies can help involve a wide variety of workers in assessing, understanding, and responding to the issues the organization faces. Such committees also provide an early warning system for organizational problems and a forum for their productive discussion. Members of cross-sectional groups should include a range of professional and nonprofessional workers.

Develop policies that maximize the benefits of expansion. A bigger budget and more staff have some obvious benefits:

- The organization is less dependent on any single worker, giving the individual more freedom and relieving the stress of having to fill numerous roles.
- More resources permit more staff training and other benefits.
- A larger staff increases the likelihood that a worker can turn for discussion and support to colleagues who face similar work problems.
- A larger organization provides opportunities for promotion and career advancement.

Policies and programs that allow staff to realize these benefits help diminish nostalgia for the "good old days" of little money and lots of commitment.

At the same time, administrators need to remind themselves and their staff of their organizational roots. Sally Dodds of HCN explained how growth can cut a group off from its constituencies. "As you become institutionalized," she said, "you start to make appointments for people to see you rather than going out to see them. Keeping a grassroots perspective means making a real commitment that comes before other commitments."

Community Problems

Even if an individual agency commits itself to playing an active role in AIDS prevention, broad community and governmental support for this mission is necessary. Otherwise, the agency will send its messages into a vacuum, or worse, spend its energy combatting opponents of AIDS prevention. This section describes some of the problems AIDS organizations and educators have encountered in building public support for prevention and some of the strategies they have used to address these obstacles.

Difficulty finding sufficient resources for AIDS prevention.

In the previous section, the problem of generating internal institutional resources was discussed. But there are limits to what any agency can produce on its own. In its 1986 report *Confronting AIDS,* the National Academy of Sciences concluded that "the most fundamental obligation for AIDS education rests with the federal government, which alone is in a position to develop and coordinate a massive campaign." In the past three years, federal funding for AIDS prevention has increased dramatically, primarily owing to the advocacy and lobbying of AIDS organizations, gay activists, public health officials, and a few elected officials. Similar efforts in cities, counties, and states across the country have also led to increases in state and local funding. The success of these activities demonstrates the value of bringing the case for AIDS prevention directly into the political arena.

At the same time, private foundations and corporations have also been educated about the AIDS epidemic and have begun to increase funding. Although most public health experts believe that significant additional resources are still needed, AIDS organizations now need to focus as much attention on how existing resources are being used as on getting more new funds.

This requires long-range planning for a variety of strategies that can help target funding effectively and support the need for additional resources. These include—

- careful evaluations of the impact of interventions on various populations and dissemination of the results to the public, scientists, and policymakers;
- ongoing surveillance of the prevalence and incidence of HIV infection to track the progress of the epidemic;
- ongoing education of political, corporate, and foundation leaders to help them understand the dimensions of the epidemic and the rationale for and impact of various interventions;
- organization of local, regional, and national coalitions to advocate comprehensive strategies for AIDS prevention;
- development of constituencies at the local, regional, and national level that understand and support AIDS prevention. Activities that can help to achieve this goal are described in Chapters 5 through 14.

This combination of scientific, educational, and political activities will help create a climate in which AIDS prevention will have broad public support.

Difficulty developing prevention programs that can reach new and diverse populations.

In Chapter 1, pedagogical and cultural factors that influence how different populations respond to AIDS prevention were described. But organizational and political obstacles also block effective prevention campaigns. The following quotes from AIDS educators illustrate the range of problems:

It is not so much that the gay AIDS organization has not tried to reach minorities as that it has not known how to try.

The Department of Health does not belong where we won't be heard. And if we're not trusted we won't be heard.

Primarily white organizations have gotten most of the funding, but they also have a lot of the expertise. There has to be a way to share the expertise, but also shift some of the money to community-based organizations.

It's a real trick—for egos more than anything else—to know when it's time to say that's not the community I should be serving and for the surrounding community to accept that.

Who can best educate whom about AIDS? How should AIDS prevention resources be allocated? How can organizations make decisions that do not reinforce racism and homophobia? These questions have set AIDS organizations against each other and undermined prevention programs throughout the country. Devising methods for addressing these problems that strengthen rather than weaken organizations is clearly an important priority.

Effective AIDS prevention programs require at least two very different kinds of expertise. One is an understanding of AIDS epidemiology and prevention strategies; the other is a detailed understanding of the culture, values, and politics of the target population. The first requires training and experience in public health, health education, or related fields. The second requires prolonged experience interacting with the intended recipients of the program, preferably by being part of their community.

One simple mechanism for helping AIDS organizations reach new populations is to include both kinds of experts in the planning process and to give them equal power in making decisions. Yes, predominantly white gay organizations have invaluable expertise in AIDS prevention, but although their contributions are necessary, they are not sufficient for planning programs in African-American and Latino communities, for women, or for young people.

In an effort to address this problem, some AIDS organizations have taken steps that have unintentionally exacerbated the problem. Examples of "solutions" that do not work are hiring one or two people of color or women as staff members and expecting these token representatives to solve the organization's problems; recruiting people of color or women as volunteers to join and support an all-white or all-male group that is unwilling to share power or resources; or abdicating any responsibility by deciding to leave AIDS education entirely to organizations of people of color or women.

More successful strategies that AIDS organizations have tried include—

- Offering technical assistance and help in fundraising to existing organizations that want to take on AIDS prevention.
- Establishing a task force on education for African-Americans or Latinos or women that has a majority of members from the target population and control of some organizational resources.
- Supporting the creation of a new group to address the needs of a population not currently being served.
- Expanding and changing the organization sufficiently so that its members and leaders reflect the diversity of the population it serves.
- Creating forums (e.g., staff training, retreats, hiring consultants) for open discussion of these problems. This solution is likely to work as a prelude to, rather than a substitute for, action.

For some AIDS organizations, the problem of reaching out is first perceived as an image issue. "Part of the reason people see us as a white, gay male organization is because that's what we grew out of," said Judy Spiegel of the AIDS Project in Los Angeles. More bluntly, a Black educator with the Philadelphia AIDS Task Force observed that "some Blacks felt that the task force was formed by gay white men to provide service for the gay center-city white boys." Often, these perceptions of organizational identity reflect not only undercurrents of homophobia and racism but also a realistic assessment of who has power in an organization. Changing the perception requires changing the reality. Viewing these conflicts simply as a public relations problem underestimates their seriousness and can hinder finding real solutions.

Competition among AIDS organizations.
AIDS organizations face a dilemma. On the one hand, most support the need for broad-based AIDS education and the right of each community to determine how best to meet that need. On the other hand, they also believe that their organization is doing critical work and needs more resources. Given limited funding, these two perceptions inevitably clash head on, and usually self-interest provides a more powerful motivator for the group's behavior.

Funding agencies often exacerbate the problem. "Sometimes funding has been done in the most divisive manner," said Judy Macks of San Francisco's AIDS Health Project. "For example, money has been taken out of health care for Native Americans and put into AIDS."

In other cases, underfunding increases conflict. "The New York State budget has made the gay and Black communities fight each other," said Lori Behrman of Gay Men's Health Crisis. "If there is any fighting, the governor is to blame. He's not providing enough to allow all these organizations to be on the front line."

Competition for funding is the most intense, but AIDS organizations also compete for reputation, turf, and political clout. Competitors often perceive that racism, homophobia, or sexism handicap their efforts to win a fair share. As one New York state legislator put it, "The big chunk of the money from the state goes to gay groups because they're more vocal, more organized, and have more access to the power brokers." The result of these perceptions is that groups often fight with each other, instead of joining forces to address a common problem.

No single strategy can eliminate this problem, but AIDS organizations have developed a variety of methods to minimize its destructive impact. These include—

- forming national and local coalitions or networks to coordinate services and lobby for more resources;
- establishing consortia to receive money and then allocate it among different groups;
- defining agendas for collective action (e.g., lobbying for legislation) while accepting that competition in other areas is inevitable;
- joining coalitions that challenge overall priorities (e.g., large military budgets) and that call for expanded funding for a variety of health and social services; and
- looking for or creating new sources of funding that are uniquely available to a specific constituency (e.g., adding money for school-based AIDS education to the education rather than the health budget).

In the long run, competition among AIDS organizations diverts energy from meeting health needs; but in the short run, organizations must find the resources they need to provide services. Acknowledging this reality without being dominated by it is perhaps the best that can be hoped for.

Problems in coordinating services with other agencies.
Competition for scarce resources, lack of any centralized planning for AIDS services, and the rapid growth of new programs have all contributed to poor coordination of services among various providers. The problem is probably worst in urban areas with a high prevalence of AIDS, but it is likely to spread to other places as patchwork funding creates similar conditions in the rest of the country. Failure

to coordinate AIDS-related services has several consequences:

- Services are duplicated.
- Linkages are inadequate between health and social services, prevention and treatment, and local and regional efforts.
- Resources are used inefficiently (e.g., a drug treatment program may be better equipped to educate drug users about AIDS than an AIDS organization).
- There is difficulty in learning from experience or generating tested models for replication.
- Some needs remain unmet.
- Different groups may deliver conflicting prevention messages, undermining their effectiveness.

What strategies have AIDS organizations used to address these problems? Establishing local or regional networks, coalitions, or consortia is one common solution. Providers of AIDS-related services meet regularly to exchange information and identify emerging needs.

In some places, the local or state public health department has initiated such a network. According to Penelope Barchfeld-Venet, AIDS education director for the Philadelphia Health Department, "Our ultimate goal is to be the coordinator of AIDS education in the city. We act as a neutral group, as a buffer between the egos of all the community-based groups." Where the health department is itself a major provider of services, a voluntary group may play the coordinating role.

Once again, a careful assessment of community needs and resources before implementing a program can prevent duplication of services. "Before you set up any services," advised Tommy Powell of Nashville Council for AIDS Resources, Education, and Support (Nashville CARES), "make sure no one else is already doing it. For example, we found some people with AIDS needed food. But we found a food bank already exists, so we coordinated with them."

Coordination in which two separate systems collaborate requires extensive communication before program implementation. "The Philadelphia schools have been very open to cooperation because we have a good ongoing relationship and good communications," explained Donald Cohen of the health department. "We met early, before the AIDS crisis hit the schools and before the first school-age AIDS case was identified. We also involved the unions from the start." In other cities, departments of health and school boards are still arguing about who is responsible for what.

Some services are probably best met on a centralized regional basis, whereas others need to be addressed at the community level. Involving coalitions or networks in setting criteria for making such decisions can establish a framework for agency administrators. Judy Macks of the AIDS Health Project in San Francisco suggested that "there needs to be a coalition that shares resources and expertise and at the same time allows people to do education in their own communities."

Difficulty convincing other organizations that AIDS is a problem they can address.

Throughout this guide, it is clear that denial is a frequent response to AIDS. As the epidemic grows, more and more organizations will need to define a role for themselves in AIDS prevention. How can AIDS educators help non-AIDS organizations take on this issue?

Define the problem in a way that is consistent with the group's mission. Too often AIDS workers assume that their sense of urgency about prevention is shared by everyone else. Few organizations, however, have the resources or commitment to add another new issue to what already seems like an overwhelming burden. By making explicit connections between the group's existing goals and services and AIDS prevention, educators can help leaders and staff to identify activities that realize both goals. For example, youth-serving agencies can be convinced that activities designed to prevent teenage pregnancy or drug abuse will also help to prevent AIDS. Another benefit of this approach is that it shows groups that the skills and expertise they already possess are directly relevant to AIDS prevention. As as result, the new mission seems less awesome. These issues are discussed more fully in the Community Education section in Chapter 4.

Help the group find new resources for AIDS prevention. Nothing is more persuasive to adding a new mission than the promise of additional dollars or other resources. Expanded federal funding for AIDS means that schools, health care institutions, prisons, and community organizations may be eligible for AIDS grants. AIDS organizations can play a useful role by making other groups aware of these opportunities and helping to submit proposals.

Larger organizations may be in a position to offer resources themselves. To help convince drug treatment programs to address the issue of AIDS, the New Jersey State Department of Health created a new position (AIDS coordinator) and provided funding to drug treatment programs to hire such a person. On a smaller scale, the Citizens Committee of New York City offered cash grants of up to $500 to neighborhood volunteer groups that developed local AIDS prevention campaigns.

Develop constituencies for AIDS prevention. Each organization responds to different players. In some cases, AIDS educators may not be the most effective spokespersons for new efforts. Identifying and educating other more influential constituencies may help to convince administrators that the problem requires their attention. School officials considering establishing AIDS education programs may listen to organized parents' groups, the teachers' union, or religious leaders. Hospital officials may find the health care workers' union more persuasive than AIDS organizations in making the case for employee education on AIDS.

By understanding the power dynamics in an organization, AIDS educators can make strategic choices about the best way to convince the group to add AIDS prevention to its agenda.

Provide technical assistance on program planning and implementation. Some organizations would consider adding AIDS prevention to their mission but do not know how to begin. In such cases, AIDS organizations can provide training, consultation, and other relevant services to help the group develop a realistic plan. For example, the Center for Community Action to Prevent AIDS at Hunter College in New York City assists community-based organizations with integrating AIDS prevention into their existing mission. By providing ongoing technical assistance, the center helps neighborhood groups plan new activities with existing resources. See the "Community Education" section in Chapter 4 for more discussion of this issue.

Opposition to AIDS prevention from political or religious groups.

Perhaps the single greatest obstacle to effective AIDS prevention has been the lack of consensus on the appropriate content for educational campaigns. As illustrated throughout this guide, almost every question that AIDS educators must address has generated conflict. In some cases, small but vocal groups have opposed clear and specific AIDS education in the schools. In others, significant sectors of the population question the wisdom of giving drug users sterile needles. Sometimes it is the US Congress that blocks funding for publications with explicit language; in other cases, the opposition of a single church leader can stop a community program from getting started.

When a society as diverse as ours confronts an epidemic as morally laden as AIDS, it is inevitable that people will disagree about how to respond; to some extent that disagreement is positive, for it forces society as a whole to consider its priorities and values. AIDS educators have addressed this problem by—

- defining a range of prevention activities, from noncontroversial to more controversial, so that every organization and community can take some action (see Figure 2);
- mobilizing constituencies that support AIDS prevention but have not previously been active on this issue;
- demonstrating the effectiveness of prevention programs both in reducing the spread of HIV infection and in addressing other related problems (e.g., STD prevention);
- clarifying the public health and moral dimensions of the epidemic so that the public at large can understand and discuss the rationale for various strategies;
- studying previous public health campaigns for relevant lessons on how to address political and religious opposition.

Social historian Allen Brandt has noted that "calls for better education are frequently offered as the best hope for controlling the AIDS epidemic. But this will only be true if some resolution is reached concerning the specific content and nature of such educational efforts."

Too often, practicing AIDS educators feel that society will not allow them to use their professional judgment in practicing health education. Educating people about AIDS without using explicit language, clear graphics, involving learners in the design of educating, or respecting differing lifestyles is like working with one's hands tied behind the back.

AIDS educators' responses to this challenge are described in the case histories in this guide. Successful strategies, discussed in greater detail elsewhere, include—

- organizing coalitions or networks that can advance the case for AIDS prevention in the political arena;
- educating the public, political leaders, administrators, and journalists about the political dimensions of AIDS and the rationale for prevention programs;
- winning ongoing support for AIDS prevention from the public at large and political leaders.

Most public health experts doubt that an effective vaccine for HIV infection can be deployed in this century. And although new drugs are being developed rapidly, it is unlikely that a cure for AIDS will be available anytime soon.

Even if such technological discoveries were to be made, it is likely that AIDS will remain a serious public health problem for decades to come, as the continued existence of syphilis, gonorrhea, and tuberculosis demonstrates.

For all these reasons, prevention will remain a central priority and education a principal strategy. As the epidemic moves into its second decade, AIDS educators will face new challenges: how to maintain support for prevention programs; how to institutionalize these programs; how to integrate AIDS prevention into the mission of other organizations; and how to maintain and support changes in behavior once the panic and hysteria subside.

As AIDS organizations begin to grapple with these questions, they have some possible strategies to consider:

- Carefully monitoring changes in knowledge, attitudes, and behaviors so that programs can choose appropriate goals. For example, researchers surveying openly gay men in urban areas have concluded that most are now aware of their risk and therefore educational interventions should emphasize building support for behavior change rather than increasing perception of risk.
- Publicizing the economic, social, and health benefits of prevention programs.
- Involving community and political leaders in prevention programs so that they feel ownership.
- Integrating AIDS prevention into the existing services provided by schools, health care institutions, and community organizations and providing these agencies with the resources needed to carry out these additional tasks.
- Sponsoring campaigns whose primary goal is to reinforce knowledge and positive attitudes and behaviors, rather than to change negative ones.
- Helping individuals, families, institutions, and communities to develop support systems that will sustain AIDS prevention activities.

In the past eight years, AIDS educators and organizations have overcome great odds to help our society learn about and take steps to prevent the further spread of this terrible epidemic. The successes of frontline activists, professionals, public officials, educators, and organizers constitute a triumph in public health history. The challenge in the years to come, as great as the ones we have just faced, is to broaden and deepen these efforts and to document their impact.

CHAPTER THREE

Educating for Health: A Framework for AIDS Educators

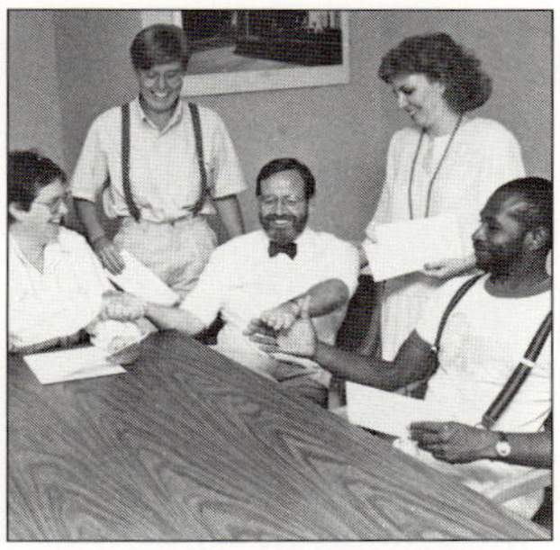

CASE HISTORY

Nashville CARES, Nashville, Tennessee

With 750 churches within its borders, Nashville is sometimes called the buckle of the Bible Belt. How can an AIDS organization grow and develop in such a climate? The story of the Nashville Council for AIDS Resources, Education, and Support (Nashville CARES) provides one answer.

Founded in August 1985, Nashville CARES established roots in the religious community from its inception. Its offices are located in a church, its executive director is a minister, and several other ministers sit on its board of directors. Churches have also provided a useful forum for public education. In September 1986, Nashville CARES sponsored an AIDS vigil in churches throughout the city. Its goals were both to commemorate those in Nashville who had died from AIDS and to educate churchgoers about the disease. Worshippers prayed, viewed films, and received literature. Organizers were particularly pleased with the good attendance at the Capital Hill First Baptist Church, one of the most important institutions in Nashville's African-American community.

Occasionally, Nashville CARES members disagreed with a particular church's viewpoint on AIDS. A church-based counseling service, for example, saw its goal as convincing gay people to become heterosexual, and AIDS as one more incentive for conversion. But according to Tommy Powell, CARES' education director, "It's better to be in contact and keep talking than to shut them off. With time," he said, "the church groups are learning not to focus on gayness but that here is an ill person who needs love and care and the Bible says we should do that."

In order to appeal to the broad range of constituencies and to survive in a conservative environment, Nashville CARES worked hard not to be identified only as a gay organization. Compassion, it insisted, was what brought its members together. The group's name, the composition of its board of directors, and its literature emphasized that it was a broad community-based group, a designation that its staff believe gave it greater authority and credibility.

Despite this approach, however, and given the public perception of AIDS and the links that its organizers had with Nashville's gay community, much of its educational work has been targeted at gay men. In fact, in early and friendly discussions with the Tennessee State Department of Health, Nashville CARES negotiated an informal arrangement in which it focused on education in the gay community while the state provided services to the general public. In the past few years, the group has run education programs in gay bars, distributed condoms, sponsored contests, and organized benefit performances of "The Normal Heart," a play about AIDS. Like gay organizations in other cities, Nashville CARES is now setting up support groups and educational workshops based in the homes of gay men.

As both public awareness and the caseload of people with AIDS grew, Nashville CARES received increasing requests for its services from outside the gay community. Its full-time executive director, part-time education director, and many volunteers now frequently speak on college campuses, at drug treatment centers, and at community organizations.

Churches provided one important route into the African-American community. Another was Meharry Medical School, a primarily Black medical college and hospital located in Nashville. Black health workers helped develop community education programs and participated in other events sponsored by Nashville CARES.

To help reach African-American gay men, Nashville CARES consulted with the Memphis chapter of Black and White Men Together, an interracial gay organization. Together the two groups produced a pamphlet aimed at this population. Nashville CARES organizers believe that their willingness to involve a variety of Black organizations in their education efforts has helped them reach Nashville's African-American community.

Other groups the organization has targeted are health and social service workers. In October 1986, the group sponsored a conference on social aspects of AIDS. More than 70 persons attended, including representatives from hospitals, schools, the parole board, prisons, and the local social security office. By applying for continuing education credits, the conference attracted many nurses and social workers. At the meeting, Nashville CARES staff made contacts that later proved useful. For example, with the representative from the social security office, they set up an expedited process for people with AIDS to get their benefits. Press coverage of the conference led to additional requests for service and training sessions. Nashville CARES has also run AIDS awareness days at both Meharry and Vanderbilt Medical Schools, showing films, distributing literature, and answering people's questions.

Mass media have played an important role in the development of Nashville

CARES. By taking the time to write concise press releases and to meet with local reporters, staff have established good rapport with several Nashville journalists. Each of its events—the church vigils, the programs in gay bars, the conference for social service workers—has received sympathetic coverage. This reporting has in turn created greater public awareness of AIDS, especially among people whom the organization might not normally reach; generated additional requests for services from new constituencies; and even led to a steady flow of unsolicited financial contributions.

Nashville CARES' successes have, of course, created new problems. Said Powell, the education director, "We often feel we're running just to stay even. We could easily use a full-time staff of five or six people, rather than the one and a half we have." As new demands for services arise, Nashville CARES, like other AIDS groups, will face the challenge of sustaining its efforts in the face of an epidemic with no early end in sight.

CASE HISTORY

BEBASHI, Philadelphia

"Will AIDS be like heart disease, diabetes, cancer, and so many other diseases where we have accepted that Black people die at higher rates than white?" asks Rashidah Hassan, the founder and director of the Philadelphia-based group, Blacks Educating Blacks About Sexual Health Issues (BEBASHI).

The answer BEBASHI hopes to offer is a strong "no." In 1985, Hassan (an infection control nurse) and others founded the group in order to begin an aggressive education campaign in Philadelphia's African-American community that could change the course of the epidemic, slowing its spread as well as strengthening the community's organization. BEBASHI also emerged in response to the failure of other Philadelphia AIDS organizations to effectively reach the Black community.

BEBASHI's messages were simple and to the point. "You don't have to be white or gay to get AIDS," proclaimed one pamphlet; "AIDS doesn't discriminate," said another. By late 1985, Blacks accounted for 100 case of AIDS in Philadelphia, more than 20% of the city's cases.

From its inception, BEBASHI sought to develop methods of education uniquely suited to the African-American community. The organization's location in the offices of the headquarters of the mostly nonwhite hospital workers' union helped to reach one sector of the Black population. This connection proved to be useful when BEBASHI was asked to develop an education program for workers in a public skilled nursing facility that resisted accepting people with AIDS. "It's not only going to be 'them,' the gay white men, who will be admitted here," Hassan told the group, "it will be people from your community as well who will need help."

After some early difficulties in getting people to accept AIDS as a Black problem, BEBASHI expanded its scope from AIDS to sexual health in general. "While the epidemic and life-threatening nature of AIDS has made AIDS education efforts among minority people our primary objective at present," explains the organization's statement of purpose, "BEBASHI also believes the Black community needs information and education regarding other sexually transmitted diseases and their serious, sometimes incapacitating complications, chronic infections, infertility, sterility, etc." This message, believes Hassan, is more acceptable and relevant to the African-American community. It also provides a framework for reaching diverse sectors of the population.

Unlike some larger AIDS organizations, BEBASHI makes no apology for targeting a specific sector of the population. "We don't believe in generic education," said Hassan. "People aren't neuter, they have their own culture, values, and patterns of communication." Effective education, she argues, must take these specifics into account.

BEBASHI believes that to be effective, educators must go to people where they work or live. Its staff offered a series of programs aimed at young people in Philadelphia's largely nonwhite housing projects. These sessions sought to reach out-of-school youth. Other programs in foster placement centers educated counselors who work with young people.

Churches play a key role in the African-American community. At first, Hassan reported, religious leaders were afraid that their constituents didn't want to hear about AIDS in churches. But as pastors began to notice that members of their congregations were dying of AIDS, they became more willing to use their churches as education forums. BEBASHI has now offered presentations in several African-American churches.

Other BEBASHI educators took to the streets, talking one on one to addicts and prostitutes and putting accurate information into the informal grapevine that spreads news among drug users. Its message for prostitutes was not moralistic: "We recognize this is your business," said BEBASHI, "but if you want to stay alive, here is how you can protect yourself."

Since many Blacks, like other Americans, learn about AIDS from the media, BEBASHI organized a presentation for the Association of Black Journalists, emphasizing that AIDS was a problem for Blacks, too, and providing reporters with accurate data on its incidence among African-Americans and Latinos.

Several of BEBASHI's organizers were veterans of the civil rights movements and other Black struggles. Thus, they acknowledged from the start that any attempt to increase awareness of and resources for the control of AIDS in the Black community had to be linked to a political campaign. "AIDS demands political activism and political responses," explained Hassan.

One strategy to achieve this end was to convince community leaders that AIDS was a problem for Blacks. BEBASHI met with officials of the Philadelphia Urban League to discuss the importance of AIDS. As a result, the Urban League's influential document "The State of Black Philadelphia—1986" included a section on AIDS. To Black city council members, BEBASHI made this argument: "If you continue to accept the portrayal of AIDS as a gay white disease, there will never be an awareness of its impact on the Black community nor will there be funds for its control." A similar message was presented at meetings for local ward leaders. By educating all levels of political leadership, BEBASHI hoped to create constituencies for the issue.

Another strategy for putting AIDS on the political agenda was to convince other groups of people of color to take on the issue. BEBASHI sent speakers to Philadelphia's Council on Latino-Puerto Rican Affairs to encourage Latino leaders to develop their own AIDS program. "You know the culture, myths, and legends of your community," BEBASHI said, "so you can educate yourselves better than anyone." Hassan has also helped to train a Latina educator about AIDS so she could spread the word in her community.

In these and other efforts, BEBASHI addressed the issue of homophobia head on. It made three arguments. First, homosexuality is not only a white condition. Some Blacks and other people of color have always been gay, whether exclusively, bisexual, or just "fooling around." Thus, to equate homosexuality with being white denies a significant reality. Second, as a people who have themselves been discriminated against and resisted injustices, Blacks should reject other forms of prejudice. And, finally, to the extent that homophobia prevents action to control AIDS, such failures will hit people of color, both gay and straight, hardest.

In its first two years of existence, BEBASHI had direct contact with more than 24,000 persons. It has educated Black leaders, organizations, and ordinary people about AIDS. It has helped other Philadelphia AIDS groups understand how to work in communities of color, and it has also worked to establish a network of African-American AIDS educators from other East Coast cities. In the past year, BEBASHI has received government funding to expand its work and has played a leadership role in advocating for more resources for AIDS prevention in Black and Latino communities.

In short, BEBASHI has demonstrated that it is possible to do AIDS education in communities of color and provides a model for those who seek an educational approach tailored to the specific needs of the African-American community.

The Process of Health Education

In Nashville, Philadelphia, and around the country, activists, educators, and health professionals are working to help people prevent the spread of AIDS. As these two case histories illustrate, educators have used a variety of methods in attempting to control the epidemic. Although most AIDS organizations share this common broad goal, they have chosen different routes to achieve it. This chapter presents educators with some choices of strategies that will help them realize their aims. Specifically, it addresses the following questions:

- How do AIDS educators choose objectives for their work?
- How do they decide whom to educate?
- What should be the content of their education?
- What educational methods are most suitable for the target population?
- How do they know if they are being successful?

To answer these questions, it is first necessary to define health education. Such a definition will help to distinguish the educational component of a comprehensive AIDS prevention and control strategy and thus to set more specific parameters for the task of educators.

Lawrence Green, a leader in the field of health education and coauthor of the influential textbook, *Health Education Planning,* has defined health education as "any combination of learning experiences designed to facilitate voluntary adoptions of behavior conducive to health." Others have emphasized the social and political dimensions of health and placed health education within the broader context of health promotion. For example, the World Health Organization has defined health promotion as "a process of enabling people to increase control over and to improve their health." Both definitions emphasize that health education involves a variety of learning activities that enable people to make significant health-related changes in their lives.

For the past seven years, AIDS educators have taught people about safer sex, advocated for more and better treatment facilities for IV drug users, counseled people about the HIV antibody test, informed people about new research findings through the mass media, helped to promote condom use, and organized in support of legislation guaranteeing the confidentiality of HIV test results. Synthesizing these activities into a definition, one could say that AIDS education refers to those activities designed to enable and encourage people to take action to prevent the spread of HIV infection. (As explained in the "Introduction and Acknowledgments," this guide is limited to discussing *preventive* AIDS education. People with AIDS have different educational needs.)

This deliberately broad definition acknowledges both the wide scope of activities carried out by those who define themselves as AIDS educators and the integral connections between AIDS education and the social and political factors described in the previous chapters. Because of the importance of these connections, the definition here emphasizes that educators cannot confine themselves only to changing the sexual and drug behaviors of those at risk of AIDS.

Choosing Objectives

Once a group has decided to address the issue of AIDS and to use education as one tool in that effort, then it must choose educational objectives. Put more simply, before deciding how to get somewhere, one has to know where one is going.

The case histories illustrate some different choices groups have made. In Nashville, the growing number of AIDS cases and the lack of action by the local health department led to the decision to create a broad-based community organization to provide information on AIDS to the general population and to groups at high risk. In Philadelphia, the perception among Black activists that the number of cases among Blacks was increasing rapidly and that other groups were not effectively reaching the African-American and Latino communities provided the impetus for founding BEBASHI.

Among the questions a group must consider in choosing its objectives are these:

- What is the pattern of disease in the community?
- What AIDS education programs are being offered by other groups?
- Which factors promoting the spread of HIV infection can be effectively blocked by an educational intervention?
- What resources are available for education?

The high prevalence of IV drug use among people with AIDS in New Jersey led the state health department to focus education on that population. In Nashville, when the Tennessee State Health Department decided to develop education materials for the general population, Nashville CARES chose to focus on the gay community. Most AIDS educators working with IV drug users are pessimistic that education alone can significantly influence a large number of addicts to seek treatment, and so they insist that drug users should learn how to clean their needles and works. And given the limited resources for education, many AIDS organizations throughout the country have chosen to target populations engaging in high-risk behaviors. Each of these decisions on objectives reflects a process of assessing the local situation and making a choice based on the findings.

Experienced AIDS educators warn of the dangers of failing to define precise objectives. "Don't bite off more than you can chew," said Anne Marie Silvia, education director of the AIDS Action Committee in Boston. "People want to do everything for everybody, but that just doesn't work. You end up doing a lousy job." More harshly, Larry Kramer, a founder and later critic of Gay Men's Health Crisis (GMHC) in New York City, observed: "For the past years, I have painfully watched as GMHC has attempted to be all things for all people, in so doing losing complete sight of the larger picture of what is happening, of what you should be doing and are not doing."

Kramer's charges, contested by current GMHC leaders, illustrate also that choosing objectives is a *political* task. To educate one group and not another, or to focus on changing individual behavior rather than on advocacy and lobbying, reflects a political analysis of what needs to be done and what can be done. AIDS organizations that fail to acknowledge and discuss this dimension of setting goals are often later wracked by dissension.

Educational research demonstrates that learners are most likely to benefit from an intervention if they participate in planning its goals and content. Too often, educators wait to involve participants in the planning process until after objectives are set. When such education fails, the learners are blamed for being passive, hostile, or apathetic. In reality, the planners often develop programs that do not address the needs of the learners.

AIDS organizations have created a variety of methods for involving groups affected by a program to help plan goals. Nashville CARES included leaders from the gay, Black, and other communities on its executive board. Health educators who provided a series of AIDS workshops for drug counselors in a therapeutic community in New York City met with management and staff before charting the objectives for the program. "What do you need to know?" they asked, and they used the answers to plan the curriculum.

Involving learners from the onset takes time and patience. In the short run, it can delay a program's start. But the long-term price of failure to include participants can be even more expensive in time and resources. Numerous AIDS organizations have become extinct and numerous educators have burned out because the people they hoped to educate perceived them as irrelevant or alien. The best way to avoid this problem is to establish a planning process that includes representatives of all groups affected by a program.

Once a group has begun to define some broad goals, how can it move to set specific objectives to come up with a plan for action? Here AIDS educators can benefit from planning models developed for other health education campaigns. One influential one, known as the PRECEDE Model, has been proposed by Lawrence Green and his colleagues. Because it is the most widely used and the most rigorously tested model, it will be briefly summarized here. Other models are described in "Resources." The purpose of Green's model is to help planners of education programs to collect relevant data, assess their significance, and then come up with a plan of action. It specifies three levels of objectives (see Figure 3). First, the program objectives describe the health outcomes and the changes in health status expected in the target population as a result of the intervention. Second, the behavioral objectives list the changes in behavior needed to improve health status. Finally, learning objectives describe knowledge, skills, or attitudes that are prerequisites for changes in behavior.

Such knowledge, skills, and attitudes are in turn shaped by what Green calls predisposing, enabling, and reinforcing factors. Predisposing factors (including knowledge, cultural values, beliefs, education, and perceptions) either support or inhibit a health behavior. Enabling factors are the skills and resources needed to perform a certain health behavior. They include health care facilities and personnel, as well as personal skills (e.g., how to clean a needle to be used for injecting drugs). Reinforcing factors encourage or discourage the desired behavior once it has been initiated. Peer or professional support and media campaigns are examples.

In this model, planners begin by defining expected improvements in health; only after charting the causal chain of events expected to lead to such improvements do they consider which educational strategy to employ to realize these goals. This method contrasts with an unfortunately

Figure 3. THE PRECEDE MODEL FOR HEALTH EDUCATION PLANNING

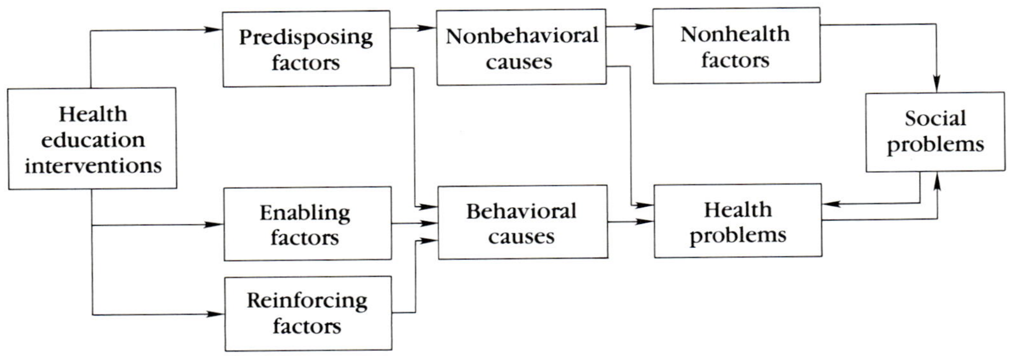

Learning Objectives	Behavioral Objectives	Program Objectives
Description of learners	Target population	Target population
Specification of knowledge, skills, or behavior to be demonstrated	Behavior to be changed	Health condition to be changed
Conditions under which such demonstration will occur	Amount of change anticipated	Amount of change anticipated
Time period	Time period	Time period

* Based on the model developed by Green L, Kreuter M, Deeds S, Partridge K: in Health Education Planning, A Diagnostic Approach. Palo Alto, Mayfield, 1980.

frequent tendency to start the planning process by writing a pamphlet or producing a video, then gearing the campaign to the available material. Figure 4 illustrates how Green's model can be used to plan an AIDS education program. Note that the planner begins on the right side of the chart, but program implementation begins on the left.

The advantage of any model, and this one in particular, is that it provides educators with a logical framework for planning. Its emphasis on health outcomes forces them to consider carefully why each activity is being carried out. Its careful analysis of the causes of behavior helps educators to develop interventions that will make a difference. But it does not tell them how to educate; it simply sets the stage for this task. It also does not in itself address the moral and social debates that the activities described in Figure 4 are certain to generate.

The disadvantage is that in simplifying reality, the model can lead to simplistic planning in which the complex range of factors affecting the success of an education program are ignored or inadequately

Figure 4. ILLUSTRATION OF THE PRECEDE MODEL FOR AIDS EDUCATION

PROGRAM PLANNER

Possible Activities	Learning Objectives*	Behavioral Objectives	Program Objectives
	EXAMPLE 1		
Lecture or film on safer sex	Explain how condoms protect against AIDS	All men who have sex with other men and who are not in a long-term (10 years or more) mutually monogamous relationship will use condoms in any sexual encounter that involves exchange of semen or blood.	The incidence of new cases of HIV infection in gay men in community X will fall from 6% to 2% in year 1 and to 0% in year 2.
Pamphlets on safer sex	Convince sexual partners to use condoms		
Support group to discuss changes in sexual behavior	Demonstrate proper use of condoms		
Condom distribution	Identify sources of condoms		
Demonstration of proper condom use	Support friends and lovers who use condoms		
	EXAMPLE 2		
Support group for women in drug treatment (also see example 1)	Discuss alternative strategies for stress reduction (also see example 1).	Women not involved in long-term mutually monogamous relationships will use condoms in all sexual encounters that involve exchange of semen or blood.	A. The incidence of new cases of HIV infection among women enrolled in drug treatment program will decrease from 4% to 2% in two years.
Training peer educators to provide ongoing referrals and assistance.	Identify sources of peer and social support for staying off drugs.	Women currently using IV drugs will end this practice.	B. Within one year, 50% of women enrolled in program will end all IV drug use.
Demonstration of needle cleaning.	Demonstrate how to clean needle and works.	Women who continue to use IV drugs will sterilize needles and works before using, or acquire their own personal needle and works.	
Small group discussion of AIDS and reproduction.	Explain perinatal transmission of AIDS.		

* Learners will be able to do as follows.

considered. More specifically, this planning model's focus on health behavior can divert the educator's attention from the broader social and political factors that influence individual and collective responses to AIDS.

Deciding Whom To Educate

Once a group has determined its educational objectives, the next step is to decide whom to educate. Related questions that must be considered include routes of HIV infection transmission in this community, who knows what about AIDS, what other education programs are being offered, and what changes are needed in order to stop the spread of HIV infection.

One useful way to begin is to list all the subpopulations in the targeted community and identify what preventive actions each can take. Figure 5 shows such a chart. The two right-hand columns require the educators to find out what education other groups are providing and to estimate what resources would be needed to have an impact on the particular subpopulation. By assessing the contribution of the desired change in each group to realizing the overall objective, education planners can decide how best to use available resources.

The case histories provide some examples of how AIDS organizations have made these decisions. Rashidah Hassan of BEBASHI defined her first task as convincing Philadelphia's African-American community that AIDS was not only a gay white disease. Otherwise, she said, "there will not be an awareness of its impact on the minority community" and no resources for preventive program will be found.

Thus, her first actions were to educate Black community leaders about AIDS. She hoped that changing the awareness of leaders would set the stage for making the community as a whole receptive to education. To achieve this aim, she gave a speech at Philadelphia's Urban League, met with Black city council representatives and church leaders, and spoke at a meeting of the Association of Black Journalists. These efforts helped create the climate for creating new community-based education programs.

Nashville CARES used churches as a forum for its AIDS education because they were a credible and powerful institution in that community. Later, when the group wanted to strengthen medical and social services for people at risk for AIDS, it sponsored the conference for health and social service workers. The conference was a starting point for building a network of concerned and informed professionals. Given its limited resources and lack of expertise in drug abuse, Nashville CARES decided *not* to develop programs for IV drug users but rather to educate the staff of drug programs so that they could educate their clients.

Just as involving program participants in planning objectives is important, so is it necessary to include representatives of affected populations in deciding *whom* to educate. The knowledge that citizens have about the power structure, communications networks, and institutions in their own communities make them invaluable contributors in selecting relevant groups in need of education.

Selecting the Content of the Education

After deciding whom to educate, the planning group must choose what they are going to say—that is, the specific messages they seek to impart. This process involves assessing (a) what people need to know in order to take effective preventive action and (b) what they already know. The former is based on our epidemiological understanding of AIDS, the latter on information elicited from the population to be educated.

Figure 5. SAMPLE WORKSHEET FOR IDENTIFYING WHO NEEDS AIDS EDUCATION IN YOUR COMMUNITY*

(1) Population Group	(2) Possible Preventive Actions	(3) Existing Programs in Your Community	(4) Needed Resources
Health professionals	Counseling patients on risk reduction; referring for needed services; providing school-based AIDS education.		
Teachers	Providing school-based AIDS education.		
Adolescents	Delaying onset of sexual intercourse; using condoms; staying off drugs.		
Community leaders	Initiating prevention programs; allocating resources.		
Parents	Educating children about AIDS.		
IV drug users	Entering drug treatment programs; practicing safer sex; cleaning needles.		
Men who have sex with other men	Practicing safer sex.		
Elected officials	Passing legislation that encourages prevention; funding prevention programs.		

* This is a process for surveying education needs; it is not a definitive list of all groups in need of education. Complete column 3 by contacting existing groups. In column 4, list estimated resources needed to develop preventive actions (column 2) that are *not* being addressed by existing programs (column 3).

In Chapter 1, the problem of deciding what to tell people about AIDS given scientific uncertainty, conflict, and ignorance was discussed. But despite the broad gaps in our understanding of AIDS, educators can in good conscience convey certain messages, and, in fact, the basic content of these has not changed substantially over the course of the epidemic. In Section II, the key messages for various populations in need of AID prevention education are discussed.

Knowing what learners already understand about a subject is important for several reasons: It saves educators from wasting time trying to teach people what they already know; it enables teachers to target their efforts on specific misunderstandings or myths; and, most important, it allows new knowledge to be anchored in existing concepts, beliefs, or values. Developing education programs without assessing the specific needs of learners is like constructing a building without first surveying the land; in both cases, the likelihood of creating a permanent structure is left to chance.

Too often, AIDS educators skip this crucial first step. "We didn't have time to do a needs assessment," reported one educator, "so we just got started using materials from other groups." One reason education planners are reluctant to carry out a needs assessment is that they believe it can be done properly only with a big budget, a long timeline, and experienced researchers. In the following pages, several inexpensive and relatively quick methods for assessing education needs are described.

A good starting point for understanding what people know and believe about AIDS is the public opinion polls conducted periodically by national news organizations and government agencies. Some examples of findings demonstrate their potential for guiding educators:

- A 1985 *New York Times*/CBS national survey showed that 28% of the sample believed that AIDS can be contracted from toilet seats, 47% from a shared glass, and 10% from handling money.
- The same survey showed that 65% of Black Americans, compared to less than 50% of the population as a whole, felt they know little or nothing about AIDS.
- A statewide survey in Illinois in 1987 found that those who most feared getting AIDS were disproportionately Latino, young, of low income, and Chicago residents.
- A 1985 national poll in the *Los Angeles Times* found that 74% of the respondents would support production and distribution of explicit safe sex materials.
- A 1987 Gallup poll showed 29% of the respondents in favor of quarantining people with AIDS and 39% opposed.

Public opinion polls provide a useful barometer of what people are thinking about AIDS. Looking at changes in responses over time is one measure of the overall impact of AIDS education. By examining the responses of subgroups of the population (e.g., young adults, African-Americans, or urban residents) educators can estimate the prevalence of various beliefs in their own community.

National polls, however, do not allow precise determination of what people think in any specific community. Nor do the questions that the news media ask always correspond to what educators need to know. Nevertheless, existing polls are an inexpensive and quick way to begin to document what people know about AIDS.

Another technique that AIDS organizations have used to assess educational need is focus groups. Developed by market researchers, focus groups provide planners with detailed information on what a sample of a target population knows and believes about a specific subject. In the usual format, eight to 20 persons are invited to meet with a facilitator to discuss a series of semistructured questions. Focus groups have been used to assess, for example, Black men's attitudes toward condoms, teenagers' reactions to an AIDS poster, and gay men's understanding of safer-sex guidelines. Figure 6 summarizes how to plan and run a focus group.

Figure 6. HOW TO PLAN AND RUN A FOCUS GROUP

Primary uses	■ To evaluate appropriateness of materials and programs for specific target groups. ■ To assess educational needs of target group. ■ To gather examples of target group's own language. ■ To gain insights into target group's perception of message.
Characteristics of focus group respondents	■ Representative of target group in race, sex, age, and class. ■ Usually paid for their participation. ■ Depending on the topic, might need to be segregated by age, race, or sex.
Role of focus group respondents	■ Expected to relate to each other rather than the moderator. ■ Exchange attitudes and candid opinions.
Characteristics of moderator	■ Not required to be an expert in the topic for discussion; strong group facilitation skills. ■ Able to skillfully probe and clarify responses from respondents without derailing discussion.
Role of moderator	■ Facilitates discussion. ■ Elicits both individual and group opinions. ■ Keeps discussion on the topic. ■ Probes to allow respondents to speak freely and spontaneously.
Resources needed for a focus group	■ Eight to 12 people in each focus group. ■ Minimum of two groups. ■ Trained moderator to lead each group. ■ Guidelines for discussion of topic. ■ Tape recorder to record discussion. ■ Neutral space to hold focus group meeting (not sponsoring agency's facility).
Advantages of focus groups	■ Format is flexible and easily modified. ■ Individual and group attitudes can be gathered at the same time. ■ Information from focus group can be used to develop quantitative tools.
Disadvantages of focus groups	■ Expensive. ■ Generate only qualitative information. ■ May not be representative. ■ Not a substitute for more extensive interaction with target group.

Although participants in focus groups are not randomly selected, planners attempt to invite people who are representative of the population to be educated. Because a number of AIDS organizations have staff with training in market research or public relations, focus groups have been widely used.

Critics point out that the method has its limitations. To assume that spending one or two hours with a small group of people can give sufficient understanding of a population to develop an appropriate education program borders on arrogance. Said Amanda Hamilton-Houston of San Francisco's Black AIDS Coalition, "Researchers run focus groups when they don't know anything about the group they're working with. If you need to do a focus group to find out what people are thinking, you're already in big trouble."

A more formal mechanism for assessing what people know about AIDS is to survey a sample of learners. By asking questions, either through an interview or on a written questionnaire, educators can take a quantitative measure of existing knowledge, beliefs, or behaviors.

For example, a questionnaire distributed to 1,326 high school students in San Francisco found that 92% correctly indicated that "sexual intercourse was one mode of contracting AIDS," but only 60% were aware that use of a condom could lower the risk of disease.

Such information can give educators precise indicators of obstacles to effective preventive action, obstacles that can then be addressed in the educational intervention. Surveys also provide baseline data that can later be used to measure the impact of the program.

Another way to understand what people know is simply to talk to them. Such a straightforward strategy can sometimes replace a more extensive research plan conducted by expensive market researchers. Criticizing a plan developed by a government agency, Amanda Hamilton-Houston noted, "We're going to wind up at the end of a needs assessment knowing exactly what we could have known if we talked to a few key people." Before developing a pamphlet on AIDS for women attending prenatal clinics, Christine Rozenrich of Baltimore's Health Education Resource Organization (HERO) spent several hours in the clinic of a city hospital. She asked women what they had heard about AIDS and what their fears were. In a later visit, she showed women a first draft of a pamphlet. When many of the women had trouble understanding the language, she switched the pamphlet to a cartoon format.

Other educators have identified community spokespersons—activists, leaders, organizers—who interact regularly with community residents and can accurately report on their beliefs and knowledge. By talking to a few such persons, the education planner can begin to map the relevant existing knowledge.

Chris Jacques, an AIDS educator with the New York City Department of Health, explained the conclusions program planners reached after interviewing community representatives in a conservative neighborhood in Queens.

Here there is the perception among residents that the epidemic is imported, that they have a "good community." If drug addicts are here, they come from Manhattan or Brooklyn. The problem is seen as getting rid of drug users and prostitutes, not ***risk reduction. They feel they have no AIDS problem here. Now that's not true, we know it's not true, but that's the perception we have to deal with when we begin AIDS education in this community.***

Without this knowledge, a totally inappropriate intervention would have been planned.

Effective use of this technique requires a careful choice of whom to talk to. If respondents are too distant from the people they report on, their perceptions may be inaccurate. Street-level youth workers, for example, may be a more valuable source of information on what out-of-school youth are thinking than the director of the local youth agency. It should also be noted that leaders do not always represent the range of viewpoints in their community, particularly when there is conflict.

No group, no matter how rooted in its own community, can assume it already knows everything about what its constituents think about AIDS. No single technique can ensure planners that they can get all the information they need to develop an education program. But any group that lacks ongoing connections to the community it expects to serve will have great difficulty in accurately assessing that population's needs. Figure 7 summarizes various strategies for assessing education needs.

Selecting Suitable Education Methods for the Target Population

Only when education planners have decided why they are saying what to whom can they begin to ask how to best get that message across. In this section, a brief review of some of the educational methods health educators can use is presented. A more detailed description of strategies for AIDS prevention is provided in Chapter 4.

Counseling. Health counseling refers to a one-on-one interaction between a health professional and a client in which both seek to develop strategies for the client to better understand his or her health needs and to facilitate behavior that protects health. Counseling includes a continuum of activities ranging from providing information to exploring alternate options for solving a problem to seeking the underlying psychodynamics motivating a particular behavior or attitude. Counseling that seeks to diagnose or treat mental health problems falls outside the professional scope of health educators.

AIDS educators have used counseling in a variety of settings. Telephone hotlines provide callers with a chance to ask questions and clarify what they need to do to protect themselves or to assess their risk of developing AIDS. Most HIV antibody testing programs provide clients with extensive counseling both before and after testing (see Chapter 4). These encounters help people understand the significance of the test, explore their reasons for wanting it, and plan how to react to a positive or a negative result. They also serve as a forum for risk reduction education.

Programs for IV drug users, like the outreach efforts of Baltimore's HERO, often rely on one-to-one counseling to help users to consider their options for quitting drugs or for taking other steps to protect themselves. In cities like San Francisco, where the health department contacts sexual partners of people with AIDS or a positive HIV test, counselors help these people to understand and act on the information they receive.

Counseling is the most individualized form of health education. It allows educators to focus on the specific concerns and needs of each client. In any given encounter, the counselor can provide information, teach new skills, or help analyze options. The emotional impact of AIDS, so often an obstacle to effective learning, can be addressed directly. A counselor can also elicit and receive immediate feedback on whether a client is achieving his or her goals. Marilyn Volker, education director of Health Crisis Network (HCN) in Miami, explained that "the real goal of AIDS education is for people to begin to think about their own lives: How do I live with this? How do I talk about this? And the most powerful—slow but powerful—part of education is what happens one on one." Helping one person to avoid infection or

Figure 7. CHECKLIST FOR ASSESSING COMMUNITY NEED FOR AIDS EDUCATION*

Questions to Answer

- What are the different population groups in this community?
- What impact has AIDS had on this community?
- What is the distribution of HIV/AIDS in this community by race, sex, age, sexual orientation, socioeconomic status, and risk behavior?
- Is AIDS prevention perceived as an important issue by community members and leaders, health and social service providers, local politicians?
- What issues are important in this community?
- Where do community members currently get information about AIDS?
- What are the common beliefs and prevalent attitudes about AIDS?
- What behaviors put people in this community at risk for HIV infection and AIDS?
- What AIDS-related services are already available in this community? (education, testing, medical care, legal, etc.)
- What other health and social services do community members regularly use? (hospitals, clinics, health departments, public assistance, drug treatment, day care, etc.)
- How could AIDS prevention be integrated into these services?
- What other health education programs have been successful in this community? Why? (prenatal care, drug abuse prevention, etc.)
- What community resources and institutions could play a role in AIDS prevention?

Sources of Information

Quantitative Data

- Health department (local, county, or state)
- CDC
- AIDS organizations
- Hospitals and health centers
- Drug treatment programs
- Professional journals
- Newspapers, television, and radio news
- Public opinion polls
- Your own research (surveys, seroprevalence studies, etc.)

Qualitative Data

- Questionnaires, interviews, and telephone interviews with
  —community members;
  —community leaders;
  —health and social service providers;
  —local politicians;
  —AIDS educators and activists.
- Community forums or meetings
- Focus groups
- Anecdotal reports from health and social service providers
- Observation of community events

Some Suggestions

- Health departments can provide AIDS surveillance data and statistics (on STDs, pregnancy and birth rates, and drug-related illness) that provide information on sexual and drug risk behaviors.
- Seroprevalence data is a useful projector of future cases of AIDS and corresponding service needs.
- A literature review may uncover previously compiled data that you could use.
- It can be expensive and time consuming to conduct your own research.
- Because each source of data has its own bias, it is important to use more than one source.
- Quantitative data can be used to justify program to funders, the community, etc., and it can be useful in both setting goals and evaluating programs.
- It is important to gather qualitative information from a range of sources that represent the community.
- Because written questionnaires can be anonymous, they are a good way of eliciting honest responses. However, they require that respondents can read and write.

* Planners may need to gather information for each population group (e.g., high school students, Black people, IV drug users, etc.).

infecting another can prevent a human, social, and economic tragedy.

On the other hand, counseling, especially one-to-one counseling, is expensive and time consuming. From an economic point of view, it is not an efficient method for providing information to large numbers of people. Competent counselors require careful training and regular supervision. They need to know what they can and cannot handle and how to refer people who need more help than they can provide. Each of these requirements demands additional resources, resources that must be available if a competent counseling program is to be established.

In addition, the counselor-client relationship is inherently unequal: one person has expertise, the other a problem. When the goal of AIDS education is to empower people, to make them more independent of professionals and institutions, counseling may need to be complemented with more self-help approaches.

Finally, counseling is a fairly intrusive method. People must be willing to seek out a counselor, find the time to talk, and accept the psychological and social consequences of admitting to having questions or problems about AIDS. Telephone hotlines minimize, but do not eliminate, these obstacles. For those who are highly motivated, counseling is probably an effective way of learning. Those who don't feel such an urgency will probably never reach a counselor. If people are forced to see a counselor (e.g., in a drug treatment program), it is less likely that the interaction will have a positive impact.

Small Groups. "We conduct safe-sex parties in people's homes," explained Leslie Kooyman, executive director of the Metrolina AIDS Project in Charlotte, North Carolina. "The parties are small, eight to ten people, informal and upbeat. The target audience is gay men. It is an excellent tool for them to discuss AIDS in a nonthreatening environment and to provide a great deal of prevention information."

Every other Sunday, a group of women married to bisexual men meet in New York City. They debate whether to get tested for HIV antibodies, whether to maintain or leave their relationship, and how to cope with their anger and their fear about AIDS. Some stay for only one or two meetings, others for months or years until, according to one observer, they have "drawn enough strength from the group to come to terms with their marriages."

In a state prison outside Baltimore, inmates meet regularly with an educator from HERO to discuss drug use, safe sex, and how to cope with the threat of AIDS while in prison.

These small groups are among a health educator's most powerful tools. AIDS educators have used small groups to present information, motivate behavior change, teach problem-solving and risk-assessment skills, clarify values, train volunteers, and provide emotional or social support.

Small groups have some of the intimacy of the counseling interaction while adding the dimension of peer support, a factor that seems to have a strong influence on health behavior. In small groups, the collective experience of the individuals who comprise it can provide a broader frame of reference than any single person can offer. Moreover, by sharing problems and analyzing their causes, members of a group can often move beyond the guilt they feel. Seeing that others share the same problems is often a first step toward action for change.

Unlike counseling, small groups are not necessarily dependent on professional participation. Sometimes a professional will initiate or lead group meetings, but many AIDS organizations have trained volunteers to conduct small group discussions on safer sex. A group facilitator who shares a life situation with group members is often a more effective leader than a professional.

Educational research suggests that, in most situations, people are more likely to learn and use new information when it is presented in a small group setting rather than in a lecture. The potential for feedback and communication among group members contributes to this effectiveness.

Small groups do have their disadvantages: They can reach only a limited number of people; participants must be highly motivated to join and to continue to attend; quality control of education can be difficult; and unless group leaders are adequately trained, they can spread misinformation or confuse participants.

In a specific group, problems can arise. A dominating or unruly member can disrupt the group. Without skilled leaders the issues that divide people—race, class, gender, sexual identity—can surface and quickly split up a group. More simply, as George Appleby of AIDS Project New Haven noted, "When one individual misses an obvious point and then runs with an illogical sequence, the confusion in the group can be difficult to counter."

Despite these limitations, however, small groups represent an effective method of education that requires personal interactions among educators and learners. AIDS educators need to learn the skills necessary to making groups work.

Lectures and Presentations. For many AIDS organizations, lectures and presentations constitute their primary education activities. Because they are a simple, adaptable, inexpensive, and practical method, they are widely used. Speakers, either health professionals or trained volunteers, present information on AIDS to a group of people assembled for that purpose. Nearly every AIDS educator can recite from memory the "AIDS 101" lecture, giving basic facts on epidemiology, transmission, and risk reduction. Such a session is usually followed by questions and answers in which listeners' specific fears, myths, and concerns are brought to the surface.

The primary goal of lectures is to present information; a skillful lecturer can use the technique effectively to convey new knowledge or reinforce existing understanding to a large group of people. AIDS educators have found that the use of audiovisual materials, personal anecdotes, case histories, and humor seems to make the material presented in a lecture more accessible. For audiences with little formal education, effective lecturing requires minimizing any similarity to a school setting.

Lectures can also help people reconsider attitudes or beliefs and begin to learn new AIDS prevention skills. Demonstrating how to use a condom, for example, may set the stage for later practice sessions.

While AIDS educators probably rely too frequently on lectures because they are familiar, it is important to distinguish between problems that arise from poor use of the technique and those that are inherent limitations.

The former category of problems can be reduced by choosing speakers carefully or by training them adequately. Inherent limitations include the difficulty of addressing the affective dimensions of AIDS and the lack of extensive interaction between speaker and audience. Marilyn Volker of Miami's HCN said that in her opinion "one-shot deals are pretty useless in terms of getting people to begin to look at behavior changes." Similarly, Judy Wenning of the West Side AIDS Project in New York City noted that "safer sex isn't an issue for a one-time discussion or lecture, but usually that's all you have." By being aware of what lectures can and cannot do, educators can use this technique appropriately.

Audiovisual Materials. Audiovisual (AV) materials include films, videos, slide shows, and other teaching aids. (Printed materials are considered in Chapter 4). They are usually used as an adjunct to more interactive forms of education. The following examples illustrate AV materials:

- In the New York Blood Bank, donors who test positive for the HIV antibody view a videotape about HIV and AIDS before meeting with a nurse for counseling.
- On many college campuses, films or videos on AIDS are shown continuously in public spaces. Students who want more information can visit the health service to talk with a professional.
- AIDS organizations in San Francisco, Baltimore, New York, Philadelphia, Los Angeles, and other cities show films or videos about safer sex in gay bars or bath houses. A volunteer is usually available to answer questions after the showing.

Because AV materials can present a consistent message time after time, they simultaneously reduce the need for expensive human resources and ensure control of the quality of information. This combination makes AV methods an administrator's joy, because expense and quality are often conflicting goals. Films and videos are also attractive because they can be used for audiences with limited reading skills, they can make a lecture format more lively or varied, and they can be used in settings where other methods of education would be difficult, such as a clinic, a waiting room, or a bar, or where language is a barrier. Their impersonality allows viewers to absorb new material without making the commitment that a personal interaction with a counselor or educator requires. Thus, they are often an effective technique for drawing people into more intensive services.

Films are also an effective training tool. They can model good communications skills or demonstrate how to teach someone to use a condom or clean needles. They can reassure trainees that talking about AIDS need not be unduly difficult.

Most limitations result from choosing inappropriate material for a specific audience. Many films on AIDS, for example, show mostly white people, reinforcing rather than challenging a Black audience's perception that AIDS is a white disease. Other films may use language that is too explicit, shocking some audiences, or too bland or vague, boring others.

The effect of a film on its audience depends on how the educator discusses the film with the audience. At a crisis shelter for runaway and homeless youth, for example, an AIDS educator reported that she frequently encounters negative reactions to portions of the film, which stresses abstinence and avoids providing information about safer sex. Because of a conservative agency policy toward sexuality, she is limited in what education materials she can use. She continues to use the film, despite some negative response, because of what it can offer the young people and because she is able to channel their criticism into a lively, productive discussion that goes beyond the film's narrow scope.

Other problems occur when educators use AV materials as a substitute rather than a supplement to interactive education. Films can't answer questions, respond to viewers' emotions, or reassure a frightened person. For this reason, any AV presentation must provide the audience with a specific link to more information and services.

How can an educator choose the most appropriate method for a specific population? No magic formula can guide the educator's choice. Rather, by carefully considering some basic principles of effective learning listed in Figure 8, the educator can plan a range of activities that are likely to achieve the program's objectives.

Figure 8. PRINCIPLES OF LEARNING RELEVANT TO AIDS EDUCATORS

- Different populations use different learning styles; educators need to understand the channels of communication of their target group.
- Each individual learns in a unique way; therefore, programs that provide a variety of methods are more likely to reach more people.
- Most people learn in several ways; therefore, programs that offer written, oral, visual, and experiential learning are more likely to have impact.
- Learning is more likely to occur when learners participate in determining the content and methods of education.
- Learning is more likely to occur when learners are actively involved in the teaching-learning interaction.
- Learning is more likely to occur when important messages are repeated.
- Changes in behavior are more likely to persist if they are reinforced by peers, family, or others.
- Effective learning addresses cognitive, affective, and skills domains.
- Learning is more likely to occur when a learner's previous experience is acknowledged and validated.
- Learning is more likely to occur when teachers and students are equal partners in a dialogue, rather than in a hierarchical relationship.
- Fear by itself is rarely a powerful incentive for learning or behavior change.
- Behavior change is more likely when educators can offer a positive plan for action rather than only a list of proscriptions.

These learning principles provide a useful checklist for educators to consult once they have developed their plans. By asking whether their interventions are in accord with these principles, they can make appropriate changes to increase the likelihood of a positive impact. The following chapters illustrate how AIDS educators have used these principles to inform their practice.

Measuring Success

Evaluation takes time so it's always the last thing we get done.

We're too busy meeting urgent needs to evaluate our program.

Yes, we evaluate our program because our funder requires us to, but all the data we collect never comes back to us in any usable way.

Quotes like these illustrate some of the negative attitudes that many AIDS educators feel toward evaluation. For service programs, the time and resources needed for evaluation rarely seem to be available; for research projects, the time and energy required for evaluation often seem to overwhelm the delivery of prevention programs.

For a variety of reasons, however, evaluation can be a powerful tool to help educators make their programs more effective. Evaluation can help to—

- demonstrate the impact of the program to administrators and funders;
- make a case for continued funding or new resources;
- provide feedback on program performance so that new approaches can be tried if necessary;

- involve staff and clients in assessing the impact of the intervention so that their stake in its success is increased;
- document the effect of the program so that others can replicate it in other settings;
- meet the legal or contractual requirements of funding agencies;
- contribute to the understanding of human behavior.

The rationale for evaluation can be administrative, scientific, or political. How to evaluate a particular program depends on who the evaluation is for and what resources are available. A program offering one or two workshops on AIDS prevention for church members, for example, requires a different level of assessment than a project funded by the National Institutes of Health that seeks to demonstrate the effectiveness of a replicable counseling and testing program. By clarifying the purposes of evaluation, planners can choose appropriate strategies.

Evaluation specialists have developed a variety of conceptual frameworks for choosing levels of evaluation. For this discussion, three different categories will be described. The starting point of evaluation is the objectives set in the planning phase. Evaluation begins when the program begins, from the left side of the model illustrated in Figure 3 (p. 42). Its purpose is to demonstrate that participants have learned new information or skills or changed their attitudes so that they can change any behaviors that are leading to impaired health.

Process evaluation refers to activities designed to assess the quantity and quality of interactions between a program and its target population. These are questions an evaluator of process might ask:

- How many and what kind of people did the program reach?
- How accurate and consistent were the messages delivered?
- To what extent did educators follow principles of effective learning?
- How satisfied were learners with their interaction with the program?
- Was the program culturally acceptable to learners?
- Did the program use its existing human and financial resources effectively and efficiently?

The techniques used by process evaluators include interviews with staff, observation of program operations, surveys of learners, small discussion groups with participants, and reviews of program materials. The goal of process evaluation is to ascertain that the program was implemented as proposed by planners and in a way consistent with realizing its objectives. It provides educators and administrators with immediate feedback that allows rapid changes in program delivery. Process evaluation begins at the same time as program implementation.

Impact evaluation measures short-term changes in learners' knowledge, attitudes, skills, and behaviors. These might be some of the questions asked in this phase:

- How much did learners' knowledge, attitudes, or behavior change as a result of the program?
- What elements of the program (e.g., small group discussions, pamphlets, or counseling) contributed to these changes?
- Did different subgroups of the target population change in different ways?

Unlike process evaluation, assessing the impact of a program requires a comparison. How much change was observed compared to what? Among the groups that can be used for such a comparison are

(1) the same group receiving the education program before the intervention (a pretest/posttest design), (2) a group that is similar in some relevant ways to the target population for whom data have already been collected (e.g., by a public opinion survey or a previous research project), (3) a group that is selected specifically to match the intervention group on relevant characteristics, or (4) a group of individuals who have been selected from the same population as the intervention group and randomly assigned to one group or the other.

In general, the more closely the group receiving the education resembles the comparison group with respect to relevant characteristics (e.g., prior knowledge of AIDS, age, sex, ethnicity, place of residence), the more likely it will be that the exposure to the intervention represents the sole difference between the two groups. The more closely both intervention and comparison groups resemble the larger population for whom this program is intended, the more certainly one can conclude that the evaluation accurately measures the program's impact. Once again, the purpose of the evaluation and the resources available will determine which comparison group is most appropriate.

Methods used to measure a program's impact include surveys, interviews, small group discussions, and, in some cases, observations. Impact evaluation begins once a program has had sufficient interactions with its participants to reasonably expect an effect.

Finally, *outcome evaluation* assesses long-term changes in health-related behavior and health status. The program objective determines the measures chosen for this level of evaluation. Common outcome indicators for AIDS prevention programs include long-term changes in drug or sexual behavior, or in HIV seroprevalence in a population. Because outcome evaluations usually require the participation of trained researchers, they will not be further discussed here. Figure 9 provides an illustration of a comprehensive evaluation plan for an AIDS education program for women in a drug treatment program.

A number of questions are frequently asked about evaluation of AIDS education programs. They are presented here, with suggested answers.

We have no money for evaluation. What can we do? Rigorous outcome evaluation is expensive, but process evaluation requires few additional resources, and every organization can do something to assess its successes.

A log book that documents the number of people receiving a particular service can provide data for measuring the impact of different outreach activities. Recording basic demographic characteristics (e.g., gender or ethnicity) of those who receive services can provide the information needed to ascertain whether target populations are being reached.

Talking to people is another inexpensive way of monitoring program effectiveness. Regular meetings with small groups of learners or informal conversations with individuals can provide valuable feedback. Marilyn Volker of Miami's HCN explained that some of the most useful evaluation happens one to one: "A person comes up to me and says, 'I learned a lot from the roleplays we did. I heard what you said, and I'm going to think about doing this or not doing that.' " Short surveys that ask respondents to rate a program or test their knowledge are also relatively easy ways to gather information.

Use of existing data or data collected for another purpose provides another way to save money. For AIDS programs based in health care institutions, medical records

Figure 9. AN EVALUATION PLAN FOR AN AIDS PREVENTION PROGRAM FOR WOMEN IN A DRUG TREATMENT PROGRAM*

Questions To Ask	Sources of Data	Criterion for Success
PROCESS EVALUATION		
Activity 1 (Support Group)		
Was group established?	Observation	Establishment of group
Did women attend?	Attendance records	At least 60% will attend four or more sessions.†
Did they participate?	Observation	All participants speak at least once each session.
Were misinformation and myths corrected?	Observation	All misinformation was corrected by participant or educator.
Activity 2 (Training Peer Educators)		
Were criteria for selecting written document developed?	Document describing criteria	
Were trainees selected based on these criteria?	Interviews with trainees and trainers; review of applications.	All trainees meet minimum standards.
Did trainees complete proposed training?	Attendance records	Trainees attend at least 80% of sessions.
Upon graduation, did peer educators meet regularly with supervisor?	Interviews with trainees and supervisors	Weekly supervision meeting for all peer educators.
Activity 3 (How To Clean Needles)		
Did all participants attend session on needle cleaning?	Attendance records	All participants attend session.
Did demonstrator give accurate description of process?	Observation	Presenter covered all points in lesson plan.
Did participants have opportunity to practice?	Observation	All participants had opportunity to practice.
Activity 4 (Discussion on AIDS and Reproduction)		
Did participants attend discussion?	Attendance records	All participants attend.
Did they participate?	Observation	All speak at least once.
Was the information presented accurately?	Observation	All points on lesson plan covered correctly.
Were cultural differences toward sexuality and reproduction respected?	Observation	Judgment of trained observer.

* See Figure 4, example 2, for objectives and activities.

† In this and other criteria for success, quantitative goals were arbitrarily set. Planners chose goals based on a review of relevant literature, reasonable expectations, and previous experience.

Figure 9. AN EVALUATION PLAN FOR AN AIDS PREVENTION PROGRAM FOR WOMEN IN A DRUG TREATMENT PROGRAM* (cont.)

Questions To Ask	Sources of Data	Criterion for Success
IMPACT EVALUATION‡		
Activity 1 (Support Group)		
Do participants in group perceive the group as supportive?	Interviews with participants	Participants report that group is supportive.
Does it increase their sense of self-esteem and self-control?	Presession and postsession test scores on standardized tests	Significant increase in post-test scores.
Do they know more about AIDS?	Presession and postsession scores on knowledge tests	Significant increase in post-test scores.
Did they learn skills for negotiating safer sex with their partners?	Observation of role plays; interviews.	Observer rates each participant on checklist.
Are they able to avoid drug use for one month? Three months?	Interviews, urine tests, medical records.	Sixty percent of participants abstain from drug use for at least one month.
Have they tried using condoms?	Interviews	Participants who have not used condoms report at least one attempt to use them.
Activity 2 (Training Peer Educators)		
Can trainees provide accurate information on AIDS to other participants?	Observations of presentations or roleplays	Observer uses checklist to document that accurate information, appropriate referrals, and proper techniques for condom use are presented.
Can they make appropriate referrals?		
Can they demonstrate condom use?		
Activity 3 (How To Clean Needles)		
Do participants know how to clean needles?	Observation	All participants demonstrate proper procedure for cleaning of drug works.
If they still inject drugs and share needles, are they cleaning needles properly?	Interviews	All participants who continue to inject drugs and share needles report that they clean needles every time.

‡ This evaluation does not include a control group; for a more rigorous assessment of this program some comparison with a similar group would be necessary. See text.

Figure 9. AN EVALUATION PLAN FOR AN AIDS PREVENTION PROGRAM FOR WOMEN IN A DRUG TREATMENT PROGRAM* (cont.)

Questions To Ask	Sources of Data	Criterion for Success
IMPACT EVALUATION (cont.)		
Activity 4 (Discussion on AIDS and Reproduction)		
Do participants understand personal risk of perinatal HIV transmission?	Interviews	All participants can explain risk of perinatal HIV transmission.
Are participants able to make informed choices on reproduction?	Interviews	Participants can describe options and behaviors needed to realize options.
Are participants using condoms regularly?	Interviews	Participants report regular condom use.
OUTCOME EVALUATION†		
Do participants continue to use condoms regularly after six months? One year?	Interviews; incidence of pregnancy and other STDs.	Eighty percent of participants report regular condom use at end of one year.
Are participants not using IV drugs after six months? One year?	Interviews; urine tests, medical records.	Eighty percent of participants are not using drugs at end of one year.
Has incidence of HIV infection declined from 4% to 2%? (See objective, Figure 4.)	Anonymous survey of blood for HIV infection at start and end of program or at six-month intervals; review of medical records.	Decline in incidence of HIV-positive cases from 4% to 2%.

† A more rigorous evaluation would require preintervention and postintervention HIV antibody tests for all participants. Participants must give informed consent for tests; documented success in reduced IV drug use and increased regular condom use are in themselves satisfactory outcomes.

can provide useful data. A decline in unwanted pregnancies among adolescents attending a clinic may indicate more effective contraceptive use. Public health data showing comparative declines in gonorrhea and syphilis in different geographic areas with high proportions of gay men have been interpreted to indicate an increase in safer-sex behavior. Public opinion polls can also document changes in attitudes or knowledge. Although such data can rarely document changes that can be solely attributed to the program, a mosaic of supporting evidence and anecdotal reports is better than no evaluation at all.

We have no one with expertise in evaluation. Whom can we turn to for help? National AIDS organizations such as the National AIDS Network; larger, more established local AIDS organizations; state health departments; and university-based researchers are all possible sources of assistance. Talking to other AIDS groups that have carried out evaluations may be helpful.

An evaluation consultant can play several roles: help think through objectives; develop appropriate questionnaires or surveys; analyze data; or take charge of the whole evaluation effort. For a one-time consultation, some evaluators will not charge, but for continuing assistance, most expect to be paid. In some cases, university researchers and community AIDS organizations have jointly applied for funding specifically to evaluate programs.

Should we hire an external evaluator? There are a few good reasons to bring in an evaluator who is not directly connected to the agency delivering the program. First, if the agency has no in-house evaluation expertise, obviously it will need to look outside for help. Second, if the evaluation is required by funders, an outsider may have more credibility than program staff. Finally, someone from the outside may be able to uncover strengths or problems not apparent to those intimately involved in the program. The resources available will influence the options chosen by an agency.

How can frontline staff be convinced that evaluation can help them? Practitioners often resent evaluation because they believe it wastes time and money, provides them with little useful information, or is used to judge them, presumably unfairly. Some of these perceptions can be addressed by education—that is, explaining why evaluation is necessary to improve program effectiveness and to win continued financial and political support for the program.

But it is also necessary to address the substance of practitioners' misgivings. Some successful strategies include—

- involving practitioners in the planning of evaluation, including the formulation of questions to be asked;
- making periodic reports to practitioners on evaluation data and asking them for their impressions of the quality and validity of findings;
- scheduling evaluation sessions in which practitioners report on their perceptions of program performance and problems;
- circulating preliminary drafts of evaluation reports for comment and criticism;
- when possible, making changes in program operation that benefit practitioners (e.g., scheduling three clients per hour rather than four and attributing this decision to evaluation data);
- training practitioners to assess their own work systematically;
- including practitioners in the preparation of published research reports and giving them credit in publications.

How can we evaluate changes in behavior when people are so reluctant to give honest information on their drug or sexual behavior? In the long run, prevention of HIV infection requires helping individuals to change their sexual behavior and use of drugs. To demonstrate the effectiveness of prevention programs, it is necessary to document such changes. In the last few years, social scientists have realized how little is known about sexual behavior, in part because research in this area has been inadequately funded. These are some principles that can guide evaluators seeking to collect such data:

- People are more likely to give accurate information if they trust the researchers. Such trust depends on understanding and supporting the goals of the research, feeling comfortable with the interviewer, and feeling that they will benefit from the interaction.
- In all settings, participants must be assured of the confidentiality of their responses. In nonclinical settings, anonymity may be desirable.
- Evaluators need to make sure that participants understand the words used to describe various sexual and drug-related behaviors.
- Interviewers need to approach the issues of drugs and sexuality nonjudgmentally.
- The overall content of the intervention being evaluated is likely to influence the willingness of participants to answer honestly. A moralistic, punitive approach to homosexuality, for example, is unlikely to encourage people to report such behavior.
- Providing needed services to participants in research projects helps to reduce their perception that they are being used by researchers who do not care about their welfare.
- In some cases, it may not be possible to collect data on sexual or drug behavior from participants. Indirect measures, however limited, may be necessary: sales or distribution of condoms, public health data on sexually transmitted diseases, the numbers of new registrants for drug treatment. Each of these sources of data limits the extent to which observed changes can be attributed to the intervention, but some limited evidence of change is better than none.

How can evaluation help us plan for the future? Careful monitoring of program performance can document successes and identify unmet needs. The Cascade AIDS Project in Portland, Oregon, for example, found that its safer-sex workshops were reaching only gay and bisexual men, changing their knowledge and attitudes about AIDS, so it began a new outreach program aimed at heterosexuals. By collecting demographic data on hotline callers before and after this campaign, they were able to judge its impact. The proportion of calls from women and male partners of prostitutes increased significantly.

An evaluation of three approaches to changing the sexual behavior of gay men by GMHC discovered that the use of an explicit film significantly increased program effectiveness. This film and other such explicit materials are now being used by AIDS organizations throughout the country.

In the midst of an epidemic, it is often difficult to take the time to assess the impact of interventions. Reaching more people somehow always seems more important. In the long run, however, every group has to justify its demands on social resources. Careful evaluations, simple or complex, inexpensive or costly, help AIDS educators to use resources more wisely, reach people more effectively, and increase their confidence that their work is making a difference.

How effectively and rapidly AIDS educators can help stop the spread of HIV infection depends on their ability to learn generalizable lessons from their experiences. Evaluation is the single most valuable way to learn what works and what does not work. It is the only way AIDS educators can develop a body of knowledge that can guide their practice.

C H A P T E R   F O U R

Strategies for AIDS Prevention

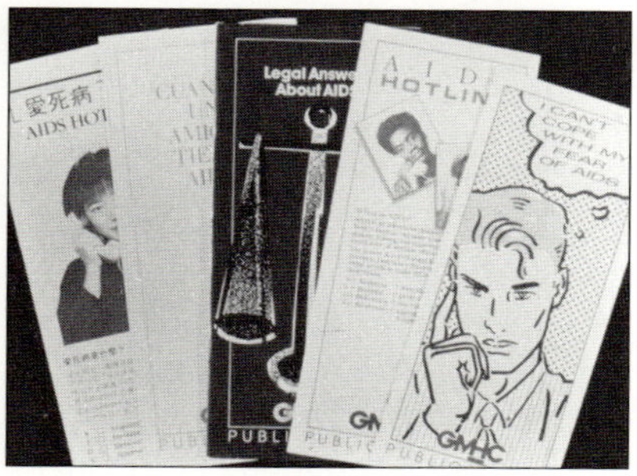

In Chapter 3, basic principles of health education that can guide AIDS educators were described. In this chapter, specific strategies that AIDS educators have used to help learners take action to prevent HIV infection are discussed. The goal is to give readers a variety of educational options to realize their program's objectives. By understanding the potentials and limits of various strategies, AIDS educators can make informed choices about how best to use resources.

Written Materials

Almost every AIDS organization has issued pamphlets for various sectors of their target population. For some groups, it is their primary activity. What can a pamphlet accomplish? What constitutes an effective piece of literature? How can a group decide whether to use materials produced by other groups or to create new ones? How can accurate and relevant information on AIDS be communicated effectively in only a few words? How do printed materials fit into a broader AIDS education strategy?

There are no easy answers to these and other questions about written materials. But by considering the issues they raise and by reviewing the experience of AIDS organizations, educators can make informed choices. Obviously, the primary goal of written materials is to provide information. "Pamphlets are a quick and inexpensive way to reach a lot of people," noted Tommy Powell of Nashville CARES. They can be distributed in places frequented by the target population (e.g., gay bars, drug treatment centers, and youth programs), they can be read in privacy, and they can provide a consistent and accurate message.

Written materials also publicize services and connect readers to sources for more information. Many telephone hotlines receive a substantial portion of their calls from people who have read a pamphlet on AIDS. For this reason, any good pamphlet must include a telephone number for those who want more information. Indeed, another function of written materials is to provoke questions and help readers relate the information to their own lives. Pamphlets also have a public relations function. They give an organization visibility and presence. "A new group's first priority," said Powell, "should be to get out literature with your name on it."

Finally, written materials can reinforce existing knowledge. For many people, it is hard to remember information on how AIDS is transmitted, what exactly constitutes safer sex, or the early symptoms of HIV infection. Pamphlets remind readers of these basic facts and provide a reference for review. To enhance this function, some AIDS organizations repeat core messages. The AIDS Action Committee in Boston, for example, prints key messages on brochures, posters, and the condom packets it distributes.

What can pamphlets *not* accomplish? They can never substitute for a comprehensive educational strategy. They usually cannot motivate and sustain changes in behavior or attitudes, nor can they provide all the information people need about AIDS. For those with limited reading skills, pamphlets that rely primarily on words will not be effective.

Effective pamphlets provide readers with a few key messages in accessible and attractive language and style. A common mistake is to pack too much information into one pamphlet, with the result that the reader never finishes. Rather than produce one general pamphlet, it might make sense to create separate pieces on AIDS transmission, the antibody test, and how to use a condom. A checklist for assessing pamphlets is illustrated in Figure 10.

Effective pamphlets persuade readers that the information relates to their lives. "Our brochures talk about the disease in a local context," explained Scott Ekbald, director of education for the Cascade AIDS Project in Portland, Oregon. "We use Oregon statistics, quotes from Oregon doctors, and graphics showing Oregon scenery." Similarly, pamphlets aimed at African-Americans and Latinos must use culturally appropriate language and graphics.

Karolynn Siegel and her colleagues at the Memorial Sloan-Kettering Cancer Center in New York City suggested several guidelines for effective safer-sex pamphlets. These included—

- an elicitation of fear about the consequences of AIDS but not its diagnosis or treatment;
- a specific description of the benefits of preventive action;
- a systematic action plan by which readers can protect themselves.

Using these and other criteria to rate 22 safer-sex pamphlets, Siegel found that a majority of those reviewed did not meet these basic guidelines.

Many AIDS organizations use pamphlets prepared by other groups. Around the country, smaller organizations distribute literature produced by Gay Men's Health Crisis (GMHC), Health Education Resource

Figure 10. CHECKLIST FOR EVALUATING EDUCATION MATERIALS

- Who is the target group?
- What do you want the target group to learn from the material?
- Is the information ACCURATE?*
  —Is the information current?
  —Is it concise?
  —Is it as unbiased as possible?
- Is the information RELEVANT† for the target group?
  —Does it reflect the values, lifestyles, and culture of the target group?
  —Does it reflect their concerns?
  —Will the target group UNDERSTAND† it?
  —Is it at their reading level?
  —Does it use their language or language that is familiar to them?
  —Is all the technical and medical jargon explained?
- Will the target group WANT† to look at it?
  —Is the layout attractive and effective?
  —Is the print large enough? Is it easy to read?
  —Are the illustrations appropriate for the target group?
  —Are the referrals current and appropriate for the target group?
  —Is it too long? Is there too much information?
  —Will it grab the target group's attention?
- Will its language or its illustrations OFFEND the target group?
  —Is it racist?
  —Is it sexist?
  —Is it homophobic?
  —Is it coercive?
  —Is it judgmental?
  —Is it sensitive to the values and culture of the target group?
- Does the material direct the target group to an easily accesible, appropriate source for more information?

---

* To verify the accuracy of information, consult reliable and knowledgeable resources, such as officials and researchers at state or local health department, health care workers, AIDS educators, research centers or hospitals, and articles in medical and health journals.

† The best way to verify relevance, appropriateness, and attractiveness of the materials is to pretest them with members of the target groups; pretest materials in focus groups or by informally talking to members of the target group in waiting rooms, stores, shopping centers, community centers, churches, etc.

Organization (HERO), San Francisco AIDS Foundation, and the American Red Cross. "We didn't want to reinvent the wheel, so we used what was available," explained one AIDS educator in the Midwest. For others, the decision is a temporary one. "We decided to reprint a San Francisco AIDS Foundation pamphlet," said Tommy Powell of Nashville CARES, "because we wanted to get something out quickly. Later we made some minor changes to make it more appropriate for Nashville."

The danger of using another group's material is that the language, context, or messages may not be exactly appropriate for the target audience. Too often, AIDS educators have distributed pamphlets produced by and for gay white men in Black and Latino communities. It is not surprising that many readers are offended or bewildered.

A sensible compromise is to use other groups' pamphlets as a starting point for producing a new piece. Few AIDS organizations object to plagiarism, as long as credit is given to the originators. A useful first step for a new AIDS organization is to collect a library of pamphlets from other organizations.

Once a group has decided to produce its own material, it is crucial to involve the target audience in the process. HERO's health educators interview a few people in the target population, produce a pamphlet based on these interviews, and then ask respondents to review the draft to make sure it addresses their concerns. HERO also keeps a record of all questions asked on its hotline and uses common questions from selected subpopulations, such as teens or Black gay men, to determine the content of the pamphlet for that group.

To produce a pamphlet for young people, the New York City Department of Health asked a group of teenagers to help them understand why their existing pamphlets were not well received by young people. Working with educators, the teens produced a piece of literature with few words, simple graphics, and a distinctly adolescent look. Both the New York City Department of Health and HERO have sponsored contests in prisons for graphics to use in AIDS materials for inmates. In both cities, inmates produced artwork aimed at arousing fear of AIDS among inmates, an approach they insisted was necessary to break through prisoners' defenses on AIDS.

In places where people speak languages other than English, AIDS educators must decide how to address these populations. In Miami, where more than 50% of the city's population is Latino and many Haitian immigrants live, Health Crisis Network (HCN) faces the challenge of providing AIDS education in three languages. Its director of education, Marilyn Volker, reported that at first existing materials were translated into Spanish and Creole, but these direct translations were found to be either awkward or too formal, and failed to consider Latino and Haitian cultural perspectives, values, and norms. Recently the group has received funding to create written materials specifically for Latinos and Haitians.

Creating printed materials for Creole-speaking Haitians brings up an interesting question regarding the appropriateness of written materials. French is the national language of Haiti and the language that is taught in the schools. However, Creole is the language that is spoken throughout Haiti. Because of high illiteracy rates in Haiti, the majority of Haitians cannot read French. Since Creole is not taught in school and is more a spoken language than a written one, AIDS educators face a challenge in trying to create printed materials that Haitians can readily understand. Pamphlets that use illustrations and symbols whenever possible allow access to AIDS-related information to people who do not read well. They are useful as well with multilingual populations.

When groups do not have the expertise to produce a pamphlet for a specific population, it makes sense to find someone who does. Nashville CARES, for example, paid an interracial gay group in Memphis to produce and print a pamphlet aimed at Tennessee's Black gay population.

Older AIDS organizations have found that their written materials must change as the population's understanding of the disease grows, as new fears emerge, or as scientific evidence changes. "As we came to understand that it was risky behaviors rather than risk groups that we had to emphasize, we had to change all our literature," reported Anne Marie Silvia of Boston's AIDS Action Council. Reports of health workers infected with HIV by splashes of blood forced educators working in hospitals to update their brochures. Failure to do so might have diminished their credibility in the eyes of the readers.

As the New York City Health Department gained experience in AIDS education, it decided to produce more narrowly targeted pamphlets and fewer general ones. It now issues separate brochures for gay men, women, African-Americans, Latinos, youths, and drug users.

Pamphlets are effective only if they reach the target audience and are read. AIDS organizations are experimenting with new ways to reach new populations. HERO produced a flyer that was mailed to all public assistance recipients in Baltimore. Several county health departments have mailed pamphlets to every resident. And in mid-1988, the Public Health Service mailed a pamphlet on AIDS to all households in the country. More such innovative approaches to distribute written materials are urgently needed.

Telephone Hotlines

Telephone hotlines have provided AIDS organizations with a direct link to people concerned about AIDS. By dialing a telephone service staffed by trained operators, callers can get information, counseling, or referrals for their specific needs. No other education method offers this combination of ready access, anonymity, and human interaction.

What can AIDS hotlines accomplish? First, they provide information to individuals so motivated to learn that they have taken action to acquire new knowledge. Hotline staff around the country report that callers continue to ask basic questions such as how AIDS is transmitted, whether their specific behavior has put them at risk, how to reduce their risk, and what the antibody test means. Thus, hotlines give information to people who are ready to hear it. Other hotlines give more specialized information. In Honolulu, Hawaii, for example, callers can hear a seven-minute taped message by calling the condom hotline.

Second, hotlines connect people to needed services. Emmett Vicars, hotline director for the Gay and Lesbian Community Service Center in Cleveland, Ohio, reported that its hotline is primarily a "referral system," most frequently sending callers to HIV testing sites. Many AIDS organizations use their hotlines to provide a first round of pretest counseling. When callers come to the testing site, they already know something about the encounter. Others are referred to physicians to assess medical symptoms, to mental health professionals to help with high levels of anxiety or depression, to dentists who provide care for HIV-infected people, to attorneys who assist in fighting discrimination, and to a variety of services for people with AIDS. To ensure that appropriate referrals are made, hotlines need accurate and up-to-date lists of available services.

A third function of hotlines is to counsel callers with AIDS concerns. As in other strategies, AIDS educators need to address feelings as well as facts. These are some of the questions that hotline operators must answer:

- How can I get my partner to use a condom?
- I want to get pregnant; should I take the AIDS test?

- I think my partner used to shoot drugs. What should I do?
- I worry about AIDS all the time. Can you help me?
- I was raped last week. Should I take the AIDS test?

To respond to these concerns, hotline staff must be able to provide information, supportive counseling, crisis intervention, and referrals. A significant proportion of calls to any hotline are from the "worried well"; reassuring these callers not only reduces their anxiety but can also contribute to diminishing the public hysteria that AIDS can evoke.

Hotlines offer direct benefits to those who call, and they also offer indirect benefits to the AIDS organizations that sponsor them. "For HERO," said Jack Stein, its executive director, "our hotline is a needs assessment tool. We look at who is calling and what people are concerned about and that helps us decide whether to make changes in outreach or budgeting. For example, beginning in 1985, more women began to call HERO, so we expanded our programs and educational materials for women." AIDS organizations also use hotlines to publicize or recruit for other programs. Callers can be mailed publications, be referred to support groups, have appointments made for HIV antibody testing, or be informed of community meetings. Because many AIDS organizations receive more than 1,000 calls a month, hotlines provide a vehicle for describing other services to a large group of concerned people.

The health care system as a whole also benefits from telephone hotlines, which provide a triage system for referring people to more intensive and expensive services. If everyone who thought his rash or weight loss might be a sign of AIDS went to a physician, the few places experienced in treating people with AIDS would be overwhelmed. By giving callers accurate information and addressing their specific concerns, hotlines can reassure those who probably do not require medical care.

Hotlines are also a useful tool for lowering community anxiety, dispelling rumors, and combatting discrimination. In 1984, for example, several callers asked the staff of the New York City Department of Health AIDS hotline whether they should fire their Haitian housekeepers. Helping the callers sort through the available information may have prevented some cases of AIDS-related job discrimination.

How To Promote Hotlines

Hotlines serve a purpose only if those who need information use the service. To solve this marketing problem, AIDS organizations have used a variety of strategies. On the broadest level, a community's perception of the AIDS organization will influence whether people turn to it for help. If heterosexuals and Blacks believe that a group helps only gay men or whites, they may choose not to call. For this reason, many AIDS organizations have defined themselves as community or social welfare organizations rather than gay or specifically AIDS related.

Other groups have set up hotlines targeted to a specific population. HERO, for example, helped establish a hotline in Montgomery County, Maryland, specifically for teenagers. Volunteer staff are teenagers, and the service is promoted to young people on radio stations and in schools.

Most AIDS organizations print their hotline number on all pieces of literature. Anyone who reads them can call the hotline for more information. Health departments and larger organizations place posters describing their services on buses and subways and in other public places. Choosing new neighborhoods in which to distribute promotional materials or publishing pamphlets in various languages provide ways for reaching new audiences.

Mass media also play a role in advertising hotlines. Some radio and television stations will accept public service announcements. Reporters and editors increasingly are willing to list hotline numbers in news reports and feature stories. Hotline staff report dramatic increases in the number of calls following such announcements.

Word of mouth is another important promotional strategy. By making sure that all calls are answered quickly, all questions are answered thoroughly and accurately, and all referrals are appropriate, hotline providers increase the likelihood that satisfied callers will refer their friends. By making sure, for example, that Spanish-speaking callers can be helped, or that safer-sex information is relevant for both gay and heterosexual callers, hotline staff can help to attract and retain users from diverse populations.

Finally, other community organizations can refer people to hotlines. By ensuring that health workers, social service workers, community organizers, and others are aware of the hotline service and can explain to their clients how to use it, AIDS organizations can make their service accessible to people who need it.

Training Hotline Staff

Some larger AIDS organizations employ paid staff to answer telephone hotlines, but most groups rely on volunteers. Thus, training these volunteers to provide consistent and high-quality services becomes an important priority. Unless an organization can offer such training, it should not consider establishing a hotline. Training programs usually require 20 to 30 hours, although some groups provide only one day of preservice training and then provide more on-the-job education.

Common topics for training include AIDS transmission and symptoms, safer-sex guidelines, referrals, and counseling techniques. Most hotlines also provide monthly training sessions to familiarize staff with new developments or to discuss emerging problems.

Some programs have developed innovative strategies for supporting volunteer hotline operators. The Good Samaritan Project in Kansas City, Missouri, for example, requires hotline staff to attend a support group meeting twice a month. These sessions provide staff an opportunity to discuss their emotional reactions to the often stressful work of answering telephone inquiries. St. Louis Effort for AIDS in Missouri publishes a newsletter for hotline volunteers both to give them information and to suggest how to handle common problems. AID Atlanta pairs a new volunteer with an experienced hotline operator to discuss calls and listen to each other answer questions for six months. When the new volunteers are ready, they begin to answer calls on their own. Developing support mechanisms such as these helps both to ensure better service and to prevent burnout and dropout. For additional discussion of training issues, see the Training section in this chapter.

Common Problems and Suggested Solutions

Hotline staff report common problems that complicate their work. These are described below, together with some solutions that have been developed.

Insufficient volunteers to staff hotline. Inadequate staffing has several negative consequences: It prevents organizations from providing services at all hours they are needed; it increases the burden on existing staff, contributing to burnout and staff turnover; and it reduces the time available for training because all staff need to be used to answer calls. Possible solutions include—

- recruiting more volunteers or recruiting from new populations, such as college students, health workers, or church groups);
- offering some benefits for volunteer staff, such as travel expenses, meals, child care, or stipends to attract people who otherwise might not be able to volunteer;
- providing services only at times of peak demand, such as late afternoons or early evenings, rather than 8 or 24 hours a day;
- using an answering machine for those times when coverage is not available;
- meeting needs of volunteers for social support, training, and recognition so that their services may be retained.

Inadequate referral sources. Hotline staff frequently complain that services are simply not available to meet the range and magnitude of needs of callers. Finding dentists who will treat HIV-infected people, lawyers to handle discrimination cases, or therapists to treat highly anxious or depressed callers can be difficult, especially in areas where AIDS has not yet been defined as a major issue.

To some extent, such problems are beyond the scope of any single hotline service. Their solution requires collaborative efforts by a variety of institutions. Hotline staff can play an important role in documenting unmet needs as a means of providing evidence for advocacy groups. Many hotlines keep a record of common questions and issue regular reports on callers' concerns.

By maintaining close ties with service providers, professional organizations, and relevant government agencies, hotlines can keep up to date on what is available and make that information accessible to their callers.

Inadequate space or telephone lines. Like other AIDS progams, hotline services often have inadequate resources to do their job. Too little money results in inadequate staff, space, or telephone technology. "We have too few telephone lines and too many calls," reported Ann Downer of the Northwest AIDS Foundation in Seattle. She also noted that lack of call-waiting equipment meant that callers were not able to get through and became discouraged from trying.

Not every program will be able to afford the most sophisticated equipment, but it makes sense for those planning to establish a hotline to talk to programs with an active service to get practical advice. Setting up a telephone bank that can expand if the need and resources grow can prevent the major problems that midpoint expansions often require.

In some areas, it might be feasible to address all the resource limitations (space, volunteers, funds) by having several AIDS-related organizations sponsor one hotline rather than each group setting up its own service.

Difficulty reaching certain populations. "We have not been able to reach Blacks or IV drug users with our hotline," reported a staff member of the St. Louis Effort Against AIDS. "Since we have no bilingual staffers," said the director of the Mississippi Gay Alliance in Jackson, "we are not reaching Hispanics or Vietnamese. We aren't reaching Blacks either." Similarly, the AID Atlanta hotline has not been successful in reaching IV drug users. Reports like these from around the country demonstrate that hotlines have not been used by all sectors of the population.

What explains this failure? On one level, it is a marketing problem. To use a hotline, people must know about it. By developing specific promotional campaigns aimed at various groups, hotline services can expand their clientele. Posters and wallet cards describing the hotline can be posted or distributed in drug treatment programs, emergency rooms, laundromats, social clubs, bars, bodegas, and high schools. Media announcements can appear in Black or Latino newspapers or on television or radio. Promotional materials need to be in the language of the target community.

The barriers to hotline use may be socioeconomic or cultural. Many low-income people do not own a telephone. Stickers with the hotline number can be posted in telephone booths in public places, or a toll-free number can eliminate the financial obstacle to making a call.

For recent immigrants and for some racial or ethnic groups, making a telephone call to a stranger to discuss sexual or drug behavior may seem peculiar, even outlandish. Such people may need to receive information through other, more familiar sources, but it may also be possible to enlist community leaders to change these attiudes. If religious leaders or trusted civic groups can describe and discuss the purposes of the hotline with their constituents, the service may be viewed more positively.

Finally, failure to reach certain groups may be caused by problems in the hotline service itself. Obviously, if none of the staff speaks Creole, Spanish, or Mandarin, callers who speak only these languages will not have their needs met. The first choice for a program is to have staff who can answer calls in all common languages. If this is not possible, part-time coverage is better than none. If, for example, a Creole-speaking volunteer is available only one day a week, promotion for the hotline in the Haitian community should ask people to call on that day. Still another option is to have written materials available in different languages. As long as a caller can give a mailing address, she or he can receive some information on AIDS. Another possibility is to refer callers to other organizations or hotlines that can speak their language.

The background of hotline operators also affects their ability to respond to callers' concerns. Bob Schoonover, director of training for AIDS Project LA, explained:

> *Now that most of our calls are from straight people, we've had to change how we train our volunteers. We're making efforts to involve a broader cross-section of people. We also can no longer assume that a caller is homosexual, and we need to be able to talk about sex between men and women as well as gay men. It was a problem for a while because nearly all of our volunteers were from the gay community and some of them had no idea what straight men and women do.*

By developing recruitment and training programs that ensure that staff are drawn from all the populations of the community and are sensitive to the sexual, gender, racial, ethnic, and religious concerns of callers, hotline providers increase the likelihood of being able to reach new populations.

Too many calls from the worried well. "I've been married for seven years and we're both faithful to each other, but ten years ago my husband slept with a prostitute once. Should I take the AIDS test?" Anyone who works on an AIDS hotline has heard questions like this hundreds, perhaps thousands, of times.

Hotline staff are frequently frustrated about how much time they spend answering such questions. On the one hand, the epidemiological evidence suggests that the risk of contracting HIV infection for people who have not engaged in high-risk behaviors is exceedingly low. Even as the epidemic spreads, the proportion of people with AIDS who can be assigned to known risk-behavior groups remains high and relatively stable. Moreover, by devoting considerable time to the "worried well," who will probably never be sick, AIDS programs may not be using limited resources efficiently.

On the other hand, the concerns of the worried well are genuine enough, and relieving their anxiety contributes to their well-being. It also can help reduce public fear and hysteria about AIDS, a benefit that makes the job of AIDS educators easier. As described previously, the reassurance that hotlines can provide also serves an important triage function, sparing other AIDS programs from meeting some of the needs of the worried well. In addition, at least some proportion of those labeled well may in fact be at some risk. The hotline may make the difference that causes such a person to get needed services or take action to prevent the infection of others.

How can AIDS hotline providers resolve their ambivalence on this question? One strategy is to increase the general awareness of AIDS through information campaigns using mass media, pamphlets, and programs based in schools, churches, and workplaces. The more the general public understands about AIDS, the more hotline staff will be able to address specific questions rather than general ones. One important goal of broad public education is to reassure the worried well and to emphasize that transmission requires an exchange of blood, semen, or vaginal fluids.

A second strategy is to market the hotline more aggressively in communities where the prevalence of HIV infection and risky behavior patterns is high. By making sure that people at higher risk of AIDS know about the hotline, providers can increase the proportion of callers from these groups.

Although no programs would want to refuse to serve the worried well, it might be helpful to develop protocols that reflect the organization's priorities. Hotline staff, for example, could be instructed to spend relatively more time on the telephone with callers who they judge to be at higher risk and less time with those judged to be at low risk. Staff must recognize, however, that a caller whose concerns are not addressed is likely to return for more services, either to the same hotline or to another program.

Difficulty of providing counseling on the telephone. Callers bring a variety of needs to an AIDS hotline. Staff can usually respond to their requests for information or for referrals relatively easily. But many callers are also in crisis. Responding to these needs in an anonymous telephone call can be difficult. A hotline's success in addressing the affective dimension of a caller's problem will determine the caller's satisfaction and likelihood of taking action.

A first prerequisite for responding to a caller's crisis is to train staff in counseling techniques. "One of our problems," reported the supervisor of a hotline run by a state health department, "is that not all our staff have backgrounds in counseling. We need to develop a training program to address this." Mental health professionals should be involved in training all hotline staff.

Second, some hotlines have developed back-up services for callers with greater needs. The New York City Department of Health hotline, for example, encourages staff to set up individual appointments with those who need more help, to refer them to the testing and counseling centers, or to invite them to join support groups run by a variety of organizations.

At a minimum, every hotline should have a list of referral centers for those who need more counseling, including places for those without financial resources, and it should establish clear guidelines for staff on what can and cannot be handled on the telephone.

Antibody Testing and Counseling

To test or not to test: No question about AIDS prevention has created more controversy than the issue of testing for the presence of antibodies to the human immunodeficiency virus (HIV). The antibody test was first licensed by the Food and Drug Administration in 1984 as a laboratory test designed to screen donated blood for evidence of HIV exposure. Since that time, proponents have encouraged testing to—

- ensure that blood, organ, and sperm donations are free of HIV infection;
- support a medical diagnosis of an individual with symptoms doctors believe may be related to HIV infection;
- indicate whether treatment with azidothymidine (AZT) or other medical interventions are appropriate;
- help women believed to be at risk of AIDS to decide whether to become pregnant or give birth;
- help women at risk of AIDS to decide whether to breastfeed or have an infant immunized with a live-virus vaccine;
- reduce anxiety in individuals who are at low risk for HIV infection yet who chronically worry about exposure;
- help scientists monitor the spread and distribution of HIV infection and track individuals who are seropositive;
- help researchers and individuals decide whether to participate in drug and vaccine trials;
- motivate individuals who are at high risk to change behaviors that endanger themselves or others.

Testing has also been encouraged to—

- identify individuals who are seropositive so that public authorities can impose restrictions or legal sanctions on them (e.g., denial of benefits or opportunities), or isolate or quarantine them;
- identify individuals who may allegedly pose a threat of HIV infection to health workers or others.

With only a few exceptions, such as protecting the blood supply and epidemiological monitoring, each of these proposed purposes has been hotly debated by public health officials, scientists, human rights advocates, AIDS activists, and elected officials. For AIDS educators, antibody testing, combined with counseling, is directly relevant to the extent that it helps individuals make informed decisions or motivates them to change risky behavior.

Before turning to the effective use of testing as an *education* strategy, the public policy dimensions of antibody testing will be briefly considered. How public health authorities (and society at large) decide to use the test for the HIV antibody will determine whether testing can be part of a comprehensive AIDS education campaign. Mandatory testing, for example, will make it far more difficult to provide counseling designed to help individuals change their behavior, because counseling usually requires voluntary participation to be effective. (Terms commonly used in discussions about testing are defined in Figure 11.)

Public Policy on Antibody Testing

Traditionally, public health officials have used screening tests to identify individuals in the early stages of an illness to provide cost-effective treatment and prevent the spread of communicable diseases. Conditions commonly screened for include tuberculosis (PPD), gonorrhea (GC culture), syphilis (RPR blood test), cervical cancer (Pap test), and lead poisoning (FEP, ZPP, or blood lead). Each of these tests provides a clinician with information that can be used to treat or make further tests; several provide information that can be used to protect public health, such as contact tracing of sexual partners of a person

Figure 11. DEFINITIONS OF TERMS USED IN ANTIBODY TESTING AND COUNSELING

Term	Definition
Antibody	A substance formed by the body as a reaction to a foreign agent or antigen.
Antigen	A protein that is foreign to the body and stimulates the formation of antibodies to combat its presence, such as a virus or bacteria.
Virus	The smallest of the microorganisms that cause disease.
HIV	Human immunodeficiency virus; a virus believed to cause AIDS.
Exposure	Contact with, but not necessarily infection by, a virus or other infectious agent. People can be exposed to the virus that causes the common cold without becoming infected.
Infection	Indicates that the infectious agent (e.g., HIV) is replicating inside the body.
HIV-positive	Refers to a person who has antibodies to HIV in the blood. In US laboratories, a positive ELISA test is repeated and then confirmed by Western Blot. Also called seropositive or HIV-infected.
HIV-negative	Refers to a person who does not have antibodies to HIV in the blood. Also called seronegative.
ELISA Test	Enzyme Linked Immunosorbent Assay; a test that detects antibodies to HIV.
Western Blot	A test for antibodies to HIV; more accurate and more expensive than the ELISA test.
Sensitivity	Probability that a test will be positive when infection is present.
Specificity	Probability that a test will be negative when infection is not present.
False positive	Test result is positive when the person tested is not actually infected.
False negative	Test result is negative when the person tested is actually infected.
Seroconversion	That time period when a person changes from being HIV negative to being HIV positive.
"Window period"	Period after infection with HIV before the body creates antibodies to the virus that can be detected by ELISA or Western Blot tests; can be as long as six months to more than 18 months, according to some researchers. The usual time range between infection and seroconversion is believed to be six to twelve weeks.
Confidential testing	Name of the person taking the test is recorded but cannot be released to unauthorized sources. In some states, positive HIV results are reported to health departments.
Anonymous testing	No specific identifying information about the person taking the test is recorded except a number selected by the person to use only when requesting test results.
Voluntary testing	Individual decides for himself or herself whether to take test.
Mandatory testing	Government or other authorities force individuals or groups of people to take the test.
Routine testing	All persons using a service are offered the test. For example, all patients admitted to a hospital.
Contact tracing	Sexual partners of a person who is HIV-positive are searched for and notified that they have been exposed to HIV.

with a sexually transmitted disease (STD) or repairs for the home of a lead-poisoned child.

The use of the antibody test for HIV differs from the use of traditional screening tests in three significant ways. First, at present there is no cure for HIV infection or AIDS. Hence, the test provides the individual with uncertain medical benefits and with information likely to be interpreted as a death sentence. Current trials of drugs such as AZT may change this situation.

Second, scientists are at present uncertain about the specific meaning of a positive antibody test. Are there seropositive individuals who have developed immunity? Are some people "carriers" who can infect others but are at no risk themselves? Are all seropositive individuals equally capable of infecting others through exchange of blood, semen, or other fluids? The available evidence suggests that a significant proportion of those with antibodies to HIV will eventually exhibit symptoms, but the answers to these questions are as yet unknown.

Moreover, the current procedures for antibody testing yield a small but measurable number of false positives and false negatives. These test errors become especially significant when screening populations at low risk of HIV infection. According to one estimate published in the *New England Journal of Medicine,* a screening program for a low-risk population such as female blood donors will yield five false positives for every ten people truly infected with HIV. Because individuals may take from six weeks to more than a year following exposure to the virus to produce measurable antibody levels, a negative test may simply indicate that the body has not yet reacted to a recent encounter with HIV. Other studies suggest that some infected individuals lose their antibodies at times.

Third, seropositive individuals or even those perceived to be seropositive are likely to experience discrimination in employment, immigration, housing, health care, and insurance. A dramatic illustration is provided by the Arcadia, Florida, family whose house was burned down in an attempt to prevent their three HIV-infected children from attending public school. Some also experience withdrawal of family or peer support and contact. Thus, the testing process can entail serious personal risk. For these reasons, screening policies for HIV infection require a different kind of scrutiny than other medical tests.

William Curran of the Harvard School of Public Health and Larry Gostin have proposed five criteria to help determine whether *mandatory* screening programs would constitute prudent public policy:

- The selected population should have a reservoir of infection so that there are not disproportionate numbers of uninfected people having to submit to intrusive testing procedures;
- The environment within which the population operates must pose a significant risk of communication of the infection;
- Knowledge of the results of testing should enable authorities to take precautions to reduce the spread of the infection that (a) would be effective and (b) would not otherwise be taken without that knowledge;
- The critical consequences of the testing and precautions must not be disproportionate to the benefits; and
- There are no less restrictive alternatives to the screening program that would be equally or more effective in meeting the public health objective.

They conclude that "it is unlikely that any proposed program for mandatory screening could meet each of these standards."

Does Antibody Testing Change Behavior?

For AIDS educators, the critical question is whether knowledge of one's antibody status contributes to reductions in risk behavior.

Public health experts disagree on the answer to this question. For example, Dr. David Cohn, coordinator of AIDS activity for the Denver Disease Control Service, asserted that "we believe strongly that people should know [their antibody status], that behavioral changes will be determined in part by that knowledge." On the other hand, Dr. Edward Brandt, former Assistant Secretary for Health and currently chair of the National Leadership Coalition on AIDS, has said, "There is no evidence to support the view that persons are more likely to change their behavior if they know they are positive." Although a number of investigators are now seeking to answer this question, unfortunately the existing evidence does not allow a definitive conclusion. Based on evidence available in mid-1989, the following preliminary generalizations seem warranted:

- Studies involving gay and bisexual men in the United States generally show that individuals who are tested report greater adherence to risk reduction guidelines than they did before being tested—no matter what the test outcome.
- Those who test positive for HIV antibodies generally make greater reductions in risk behavior than those who test negative.
- Studies comparing behavior change between those who choose to be tested and those who do not show contradictory results.
- Some significant proportion of those who test positive experience depression, isolation, and serious anxiety after learning the results.
- Different populations respond to the antibody test differently.

Preliminary research results and anecdotal reports from clinicians suggest that, after learning the results of the test, some IV drug users may be more likely to increase risk behavior (e.g., drug use and unprotected intercourse) than are gay men. Dr. Frank Cancellieri and his colleagues at the Downstate SUNY Health Science Center in Brooklyn, for example, reported that, based on their study of 57 pregnant women in drug treatment programs, "the testing process can precipitate serious psychiatric problems, principally in the form of increased drug use which can have a devastating medical and psychiatric impact in this group of already emotionally impaired individuals." As new groups such as adolescents and mentally retarded people become candidates for HIV testing, it is important to ensure *before* testing begins that the process will in fact benefit individuals.

Most AIDS workers who participate in testing programs emphasize the critical importance of pretest and posttest counseling. For example, Dr. Peter Selwyn and his colleagues at Montefiore Medical Center in the Bronx concluded that the behavior change observed among clients in a drug treatment program was due to education and counseling rather than to knowledge of antibody status. Similarly, David Miller and his colleagues at the National AIDS Counseling Training Unit in London reported that "personal knowledge of antibody state seems to be a less important motivator for behavioral change than sustained and consistent counseling from various sources."

Peter Goldblum and Neil Seymour of San Francisco's AIDS Project emphasized the importance of counseling for sustaining behavioral changes. "The person who feels that it is necessary to take the test in order to be shocked into compliance with risk guidelines," they wrote, "may need to continue seeing a counselor to accomplish this goal realistically. Shock value is only effective in the short term, and long-term strategies are essential with AIDS risk prevention."

Guidelines for Antibody Testing and Counseling

Given the importance of counseling, how can AIDS educators contribute to the development of effective testing and counseling programs? The following guidelines focus on the *educational* impact of testing and counseling programs. They do not consider the full range of ethical, legal, and medical questions that staff of such programs must address.

Counseling is most effective when people are already knowledgeable about AIDS; therefore, general public AIDS education is an important prerequisite for efficient use of antibody testing and counseling programs. The more people know about AIDS, the better able they are to make informed choices about whether to take the HIV antibody test and to interpret the results. In addition, when clients are better informed, counselors can focus on individual concerns and a specific plan for risk reduction rather than simply providing basic information.

For these reasons, many testing programs seek to provide some education *before* an appointment for testing. Telephone hotlines, for example, often provide facts on AIDS and the antibody test, then offer an appointment for additional counseling and possible testing. In STD clinics run by the New York City Department of Health, AIDS educators give a short talk on AIDS in the clinic waiting room, then offer to meet privately with anyone who wants more information on the test. Other groups distribute brochures describing the test, listing a telephone number or clinic where more information is available.

AIDS counselors require careful training and close supervision. "In that short time you spend with a client talking about AIDS and the test," reported one AIDS counselor working at an anonymous test site, "anything can come up—feelings about sex and drugs, suicide, fear of being rejected by a lover or family, past experiences of sexual abuse; it can get very intense." Preparing counselors to deal with these intense experiences requires carefully planned training, a requirement often overlooked by those advocating widespread testing.

According to Dr. Stephen Joseph, Health Commissioner of New York City, "the biggest constraint to increasing voluntary testing is the lack of trained counselors." AIDS organizations that support testing as a preventive strategy need to develop the capacity to train staff to provide adequate counseling. Competent counselors need to know the natural history of HIV infection, the significance of the antibody test, and the behaviors needed to reduce the risk of HIV infection. In addition, they need to be able to elicit information, provide nonjudgmental counseling, refer to other services, and prepare clients to protect themselves against any discrimination they may encounter. Figure 12 lists the skills and knowledge counselors need, and Figure 13 provides an outline for a training program for counselors.

Counselors also need professional supervision. They must be able to discuss difficult cases, receive feedback on their counseling, and get support for the emotional drain that AIDS counseling entails. Lack of such supervision can lead to poor services or staff burnout and subsequent high turnover. Counselors need to find out what clients already know and how they feel about AIDS.

Counselors usually have only a short time, typically 10 to 60 minutes, to achieve many objectives, such as a decision on testing, a plan for risk reduction, or a decision on the need for referrals. Therefore,

Figure 12. OBJECTIVES OF A FIVE-DAY TRAINING PROGRAM FOR AIDS COUNSELORS

At the end of this training, participants will be able to—

- provide their clients with accurate and relevant information on AIDS;
- assist clients in taking action to reduce their risks of HIV infection;
- counsel those who seek information on the HIV antibody test and help clients assess advantages and disadvantages of the antibody test;
- provide supportive counseling for those who need it;
- assist clients in making informed choices about reproduction in the light of current knowledge of HIV infection;
- provide referrals for needed medical, legal, social, or other services.

it is crucial that the available time be used effectively. This precludes "cookbook" counseling or didactic presentations. These are some of the questions that counselors have found helpful to begin the process:

- What brings you here today?
- What makes you think you might be at risk for AIDS?
- How do you plan to use the information the test provides?
- What do you think the test can tell you?
- What do you know about how AIDS is passed on?

By listening carefully to the answers, a counselor can assess the client's knowledge, level of anxiety, and need for services. A counselor can also pick up on the client's language about sex, drugs, relationships, health, and disease and respond in a way that ensures real communication.

Counselors must be prepared to raise issues such as drug use and sexual behavior in a way that encourages clients to talk. Too often, according to sex educator Michael Carrera, health professionals believe that there is a "correct" way to talk about sex and an incorrect or "vulgar" way. "If you talk about insertive anogenital intercourse to teens," he said, "they don't know what you're talking about." Language is power, and especially when talking about sex, the words that are used can reinforce or break down the professional/client hierarchy.

Trust, or *confianza,* is an essential prerequisite for effective counseling, said Ruth Rodriguez of the Hispanic AIDS Forum in New York City. Choosing a language that both counselor and client can use comfortably is a first step in establishing trust. "I often ask a client: Should we use street language or doctor's office talk?" reported one AIDS counselor.

Nonverbal communication is as important as words. The raised eyebrow at the mention of homosexual activity or the wrinkled nose when drug use is discussed can quickly shut the door to further discussion. Nonverbal gestures can also carry different messages in different cultures, which makes a cross-cultural education for counselors important.

To make the counseling experience an opportunity for risk reduction education, the question of testing must be presented as one preventive strategy among many. If counselors discuss with their clients only the test, they lose the chance to make a more significant contribution—to help clients change the behaviors that put them at risk of HIV infection. By developing counseling protocols that ensure that risk reduction information is presented and discussed with all clients, testing programs increase their educational impact. Figure 14 illustrates one such protocol, listing the topics counselors should cover.

Figure 13. OUTLINE OF A FIVE-DAY TRAINING PROGRAM FOR AIDS COUNSELORS*

Day One	
9:00 - 9:30	Pretest
9:30 - 10:00	Introductions
10:00 - 10:15	Orientation/preview
10:15 - 12:30	An Overview: What You and Your Clients Need To Know About AIDS and HIV Infection
12:30 - 1:30	Lunch
1:30 - 2:30	Counseling Techniques: HIV Infection and Risk Reduction
2:30 - 3:30	Role Plays: Counseling Clients About AIDS and HIV Infection
3:30 - 3:45	Break
3:45 - 5:00	Activity: Understanding Obstacles to Behavior Change

Day Two	
9:00 - 10:00	HIV Infection and Discrimination
10:00 - 10:45	Small Group Discussion: Protecting Client Confidentiality
10:45 - 11:00	Break
11:00 - 12:30	AIDS and Sexuality
12:30 - 1:30	Lunch
1:30 - 3:00	Activities and Discussion: Safer Sex and Risk Reduction
3:00 - 3:15	Break
3:15 - 4:30	Role Plays: Counseling Clients About Sexuality and Risk Reduction

Day Three	
9:00 - 10:00	Race, Culture, Class, and Values: How They Affect the Counseling Interaction
10:00 - 10:30	Discussion: Factors That Influence the Interaction Between Client and Counselor
10:30 - 10:45	Break
10:45 - 12:00	Activity: Redesigning Our Agencies
12:00 - 1:00	Lunch
1:00 - 3:00	AIDS and Drugs: Counseling and Education
3:00 - 3:15	Break
3:15 - 4:30	Role Plays: Counseling Clients About Drugs

Day Four	
9:00 - 10:00	Women, Reproduction, and AIDS
10:00 - 10:45	Case Study and Role Plays: Counseling Women About HIV Infection
10:45 - 11:00	Break
11:00 - 12:00	Overview: The HIV Antibody Test
12:00 - 12:30	Counseling Clients When Time Is Limited
12:30 - 1:30	Lunch
1:30 - 2:30	Counseling Techniques: Pretest Counseling
2:30 - 3:00	Discussion: Issues and Problems of Pretest Counseling
3:00 - 3:15	Break
3:15 - 4:30	Role Plays: Counseling Clients About the HIV Test and Pretest Counseling

Day Five	
9:00 - 10:00	Counseling Techniques: Posttest Counseling
10:00 - 11:00	Role Plays: Helping Clients Cope With the Knowledge of Their Antibody Status
11:00 - 11:15	Break
11:15 - 12:30	Small Group Discussion: Integrating AIDS Education and Counseling Into Your Work Setting
3:00 - 3:30	Summary and Evaluation
3:30 - 4:00	Posttest

* The purpose of this training is to realize the objectives listed in Figure 12.

Figure 14. PROTOCOL FOR PRETEST AND POSTTEST COUNSELING

Pretest Questions

1. Why are you taking the test now?
2. What does the HIV test mean to you?
3. What does a positive result mean?
4. What does a negative result mean?
5. What's the difference between a positive HIV test and AIDS?
6. Do you know what your personal risk is? What can you do to make those behaviors safer?
7. What specifically will you do if you're positive?
8. What specifically will you do if you're negative?
9. Do you plan on telling your partner of the result?
10. Do you plan on telling your partner of your risk?
11. Do you plan on practicing safer sex? If so, how?
12. Do you plan on stopping IV use or doing safer drug use?
13. What are your barriers and motivators to risk reduction?
14. How have you handled stressful situations in the past?

Pretest Counseling Assessment

1. Does the patient have an accurate understanding of the significance of the test?
2. Is the patient rational?
3. Does the person's level of anxiety get in the way of adequate communication about testing?
4. Is this person potentially at risk for hurting himself or herself? Others?
5. Do you believe that the testing will interfere with the individual's capacity to develop and/or maintain healthy maintenance actions?
6. Do you believe that the individual is taking all the positive action to secure his or her health now? Specify.
7. Identify barriers to individual implementing or consistently using risk reduction (if applicable). Specify resource for addressing these problems.
8. Do you believe that the individual could handle the test results and might benefit from the information? If not, why? If so, how?

Figure 14. PROTOCOL FOR PRETEST AND POSTTEST COUNSELING (cont.)

Posttest Counseling Assessment

1. Does client understand the meaning of the test?
   ______ Infected with HIV virus.
   ______ Assume able to transmit.
   ______ Possible future health status includes healthy, symptomatic, ARC, AIDS.
   Comments?

2. Does client understand need for risk reduction?
   ______ Preventing further exposure, including minimizing repeat exposure to virus or its variations.
   ______ Preventing transmission to others.
   Comments?

3. Does client understand risk reduction techniques?

   Safer sex:
   ______ Avoiding ingestion or transmission of semen.
   ______ Using condoms properly.
   ______ Limiting contact with vaginal secretions.

   Needle use:
   ______ Avoiding needle sharing.
   ______ Cleaning needles properly.
   ______ Getting drug treatment for addiction.

   Comments?

4. Does client plan on making lifestyle changes?
   ______ Safer sex.
   ______ Safer/no drug abuse.
   ______ Health maintenance.
   —diet
   —stress reduction
   —exercise
   —regular health care
   ______ Using special resources to implement/reinforce change.
   Comments?

Figure 14. PROTOCOL FOR PRETEST AND POSTTEST COUNSELING (cont.)

Posttest Counseling Assessment

5. Does client know how to protect his or her confidentiality?
   ______ Avoiding discrimination in work, housing, insurance.
   ______ Knowing he or she has a right not to tell.
   ______ Telling medical professionals in a safe way.
   Comments?

6. Does client know how to tell past and present sexual or needle-sharing partners?
   ______ Knows strategies for sharing information in a way that protects both parties.
   ______ Knows that counselor will accept partner referral and do joint or individual counseling.
   Comments?

7. Does client have an adequate support system?
   ______ Can discuss this with a close friend.
   ______ Can discuss this with a lover or spouse.
   ______ Can discuss this with a family member.
   ______ Involved with counseling or support group.
   ______ Involved with religious organization.
   Comments?

8. Assessment of need for support. Referrals given:
   ______ Health.
   ______ Social service.
   ______ Emotional support.
   ______ Risk reduction services.
   ______ Other.

9. Is follow-up appointment necessary?

   Concerning what issues?

   Comments?

Each client should leave the testing and counseling encounter with a specific plan for risk reduction. Some programs present risk reduction information in the pretest counseling, others leave it for the posttest session, and still others discuss risk reduction in both sessions. Whatever the timing, clients should take away from the experience an understanding of which, if any, of their current activities put them or their partners at risk of HIV infection and what steps they can take to reduce or eliminate these risks.

Such a plan must be individualized; for the drug addict unable or unwilling to stop using drugs, for example, information on how to clean injection paraphernalia must be presented. For the man who says he cannot tell his wife about his other partners, a counselor can explore how to bring up the issue of condom use.

The information and skills a counselor provides are worthwhile only to the extent that a client can use them. It is the *counselor's* responsibility to maximize this likelihood. The specific actions a counselor can take include involving the client's lover, family, or friends in the prevention plan, helping the client to identify the benefits of change, looking for positive reinforcers of risk reduction behavior, and connecting the client to community groups or professional agencies that can support changes in behavior.

Counselors must be able to identify clients in need of more education, psychiatric help, or other services and to provide appropriate referral services. Most testing and counseling programs do not have the resources to meet the entire range of needs that come up in the encounter. Yet any ethical program must be able to provide clients with services to address the problems its counselors uncover.

Common reactions to a positive antibody test are depression, grief, anxiety, and social isolation. Counselors can sometimes elicit the potential for problems *before* the test and help clients to seek preventive counseling. Many programs run ongoing support groups for those who have tested HIV positive; counselors in these programs can make this service available to all clients who want it. Some clients will need more education than the one or two counseling sessions can provide. Robert Stemple of the University of California at San Francisco observed that some individuals continue to engage in high-risk activities and require special educational interventions. A self-help group may be an appropriate referral for such people.

Counselors must also be prepared to respond adequately to reports of rape, sexual abuse, suicide attempts, serious anxiety about health, and other such issues.

Counselors must warn clients of the potential negative consequences of antibody testing and prepare them to minimize these problems. "Clinically, knowing your antibody status might be somewhat useful," admitted Mark Senak, director of legal services for GMHC, "but practically it can ruin your life." People considering being tested for HIV need to know that some have lost jobs, housing, health insurance, friends, and lovers as a result of the test. Even though much discrimination is illegal, only those with the resources to seek legal protection can remedy these wrongs. No laws protect the individual from discrimination by family and friends who fear contact with someone who is or who is believed to be HIV infected.

By carefully explaining who will have access to test results and by exploring with the clients in advance whom they will discuss the results with, counselors can help a client to make informed choices.

The final decision on whether to be tested is the client's. According to Lawrence Green, former director of the Center for Health Promotion Research and Development at the University of Texas, and his colleagues, the defining characteristic of health education is the "voluntary participation of the consumer in determining his or her own health practices." They argue that this is not merely a philosophical tenet, but is based on the "overwhelming" evidence that the "durability of cognitive and behavioral changes is proportional to the degree of active rather than passive participation of the learner."

Policies on HIV testing will be determined by a variety of political and scientific factors. To the extent that testing is designed to be an *education* strategy, however, AIDS educators must insist that participation be voluntary.

National and institutional policies define one dimension of clients' freedom to make choices. Counselors' attitudes and behaviors shape another dimension. It is easy to understand why counselors might feel some clients *should* be tested—the drug-addicted woman who does not use birth control, the gay male prostitute, or the former IV drug user about to enter a new relationship. But as Green noted, the commitment to voluntary choice is both philosophical and practical. The client who perceives a counselor pushing him or her to take an undesired action is less likely to be open to the information that could make a greater long-term difference than the test itself.

Mass Media

According to national public opinion polls, the people of the United States learn more about AIDS from the mass media than from any other source. No other channel of communications so pervades our society as television, radio, magazines, and newspapers. And no other institutions—not schools, not hospitals, not churches—so dominate the day-to-day work of health educators. "The day the story hit the media about the three health workers infected with HIV from blood splashes, my telephone never stopped ringing," reported Jeanne Kalinoski, AIDS educator for the employees of New York City's Bellevue Hospital. "I spend more than half my time correcting misinformation spread by sensational news coverage," said another AIDS educator. For all these reasons, health educators need to understand how mass media affect the public and how they can use the media to encourage preventive action.

Advantages and Disadvantages of Mass Media

What can mass media accomplish? For one thing they can reach millions of people. A story covered by the evening network news on all three channels will reach 50 million people; if all daily newspapers report a story, 75 million homes can be reached overnight. For organizations able to work on a national level, media can be economical. According to Art Ulene, producer of "Feeling Fine" and commentator on NBC's "Today" show, one can reach 50 million people with a message that may cost only $3,000 to develop. This same message can be delivered repeatedly, reinforcing it over time and reaching people who cannot be present all at once.

What the media can do best is present information. The public's understanding of how AIDS is transmitted, who is affected, and how to protect oneself depends in large part on media coverage. Public opinion polls that show increasingly accurate understanding about AIDS suggest that the media have played a positive role in transmitting information. Repetition of basic facts about AIIDS in news reports, public service announcements, and talk shows also reinforces information people already know. Like pamphlets, mass media offer the potential (if not always the reality) for strict control of the quality of the information going out to the public.

Media messages can also encourage people to seek more information about AIDS. Nathan Maccoby, associate director of the Center for Research in Disease Prevention at Stanford University, noted that television and radio "can play a major role in getting people to pay attention when information in greater detail is available." Marilyn Volker, education director of HCN in Miami, called media "the connector, the first stimulus around safer sex and condom use. Then people need to know where to go for further information." Many AIDS organizations use the media to publicize their services. "If our phone number is shown three times on a one-hour AIDS show on television, we can expect 70 to 100 phone calls," reported Garry Anderson, executive director of the AIDS Project in Portland, Maine.

Media also help to set the public agenda on AIDS. Said Maccoby of Stanford University, the media "can take an issue that's on the back burner and put it on the front burner. They set the agenda for people's ideas, thoughts, discussions, plans, and actions." AIDS is a national political issue in large part because the media have made it one.

One specific way to use the media's agenda-setting power is to target legislators. "When a politician knows the whole community is hearing what he has done, it's the most effective way of changing his behavior," observed Tony Schwartz, a media consultant for presidential candidates, corporations, and national health organization. By encouraging media coverage of expenditures on AIDS, gay activists in New York City, San Francisco, and Los Angeles helped convince city governments to appropriate more resources for prevention and treatment.

Finally, because they reach almost all sectors of the population, newspapers, radio, and television can be used to bring messages to groups hard to reach by any other method. Homosexual men who are "in the closet," married bisexual men, the drug user who shoots up once a month—almost all these are exposed to the mass media, which may provide the first message that informs them they are at risk of HIV infection. Even IV drug users, a group frequently believed to be isolated from mainstream society, report that television, newspapers, and radio are important sources of AIDS information. Since broadcast journalism does not require literacy and many daily newspapers are written at an eighth-grade reading level, media can also reach those with limited reading skills.

Some of the educational advantages of mass media are also disadvantages. Because of their large audience, media can spread misinformation throughout the population. The emphasis on the handful of children with AIDS attending public schools, for example, obscured the fact that most children with AIDS die before their third birthday. Sensationalized reports of the discovery of HIV in saliva contributed to inaccurate perceptions of the syndrome's contagiousness. AIDS organizations that operate telephone hotlines claim that media coverage of AIDS generates a significant proportion of calls from people who misperceive their risk or are unduly alarmed.

How the mass media cover AIDS has also contributed to obstacles that educators face. Editors and reporters tend to develop "frames" on stories—simplified images that can be used to quickly transmit ideas. The frames that have been used to cover AIDS—the "gay plague," "innocent victims," the infected prostitute who continues to sell his or her body—have reinforced homophobia, downplayed the toll of AIDS on African-Americans and Latinos, fanned hysteria, and helped create a climate in which politicians can promote repressive but ineffective policies. For this reason, many AIDS educators see their task as countering the media's images of AIDS, rather than working with reporters. Some of this negative attitude may be based on educators' misunderstanding of the media's role. "Often we rely too much on media," said Marilyn Volker of HCN in Miami, "and because we rely too much, we bad-mouth media."

Media are not particularly effective by themselves in changing deep-rooted behavior. "By and large, television cultivates resistance to change," observed George Gerbner, dean of the Annenberg School of Communication at the University of Pennsylvania. It is a conservative social institution that seeks not to offend or alienate significant sectors of the population. The refusal of most television stations to broadcast condom commercials illustrates this attitude.

Usually the media are too impersonal to address the deeply held beliefs that influence behavior. "I don't think media coverage is ever sufficient" to inspire fundamental changes in sexual practices and drug use, noted Lawrence Green.

Mass media also cannot elicit detailed feedback from learners, they cannot stimulate dialogue, and they cannot build personal support networks. Most important, as with any other strategy, they are not a substitute for a comprehensive health education program. Despite these limitations, mass media have had profound influence on how the American people view sexuality and drugs. Whether the media's desire to use public interest in sex and drugs to sell products or increase circulation can be translated into effective AIDS prevention messages remains to be seen.

With this backdrop, what recommendations can be suggested for AIDS educators seeking to use the media effectively? The following tips are based on interviews with educators and reporters and reviews of relevant literature.

Recommendations for Effective Use of Media To Educate People About AIDS

Learn what is considered newsworthy. The average newspaper receive 200 press releases a day; unless the editors see something that grabs their attention, most end up in the wastebasket. Editors want something that is new, of human interest, or somehow important to their readers. Issuing a press release every week wastes the time for the staff person who writes it and the editor who reads it.

Roger Burr, program director for STD and AIDS education in the Wyoming State Department of Health, reported that an occasional news conference worked better than frequent press releases. "With individual news releases," he said, "the media pick and choose which they will use," but "we have had a very good response with a news conference. We explain our program plans and then answer reporters' questions."

AIDS educators can learn what interests reporters by talking to them, by following coverage in local media, and by presenting them with a few different angles on potential stories—for example, a local perspective, a human interest side, or a political dimension.

Do not exaggerate or lie to journalists. In their eagerness to get a message out or to put their organizations in a favorable light, staff of AIDS organizations will sometimes stretch the truth. The results can be disastrous. For example, Secretary of Health and Human Services Margaret Heckler's 1984 announcement at a press conference that a vaccine would be "ready for testing" in two years further discredited the government she served.

Credibility is a vital asset for public health workers. If reporters know a source will always give accurate information, they will come back to check facts, elicit quotes, or look for story ideas. "We have developed a positive relationship with the media, building credibility; so now they turn to us first for information and guidance," reported Scott Ekblad of the Cascade AIDS Project in Oregon.

But telling the truth is not enough. AIDS workers also need to learn how to get their message across in a few words that are also accurate. Rehearsing the two or three key ideas that the AIDS organization wants to get out helps some people to prepare for encounters with reporters.

Include reporters, editors, and publishers as a target population to be educated. In 1983, early in the AIDS epidemic, the Philadelphia AIDS Task Force decided that accurate media coverage of th epidemic would help to both educate the public and build the organization. So they identified a reporter on a daily newspaper and began to educate him. They sent him a file of articles on AIDS from scientific journals. They escorted him on a visit to gay bars and bathhouses so he could better understand gay culture. His subsequent series on AIDS not only brought thousands of Philadelphians their first news of the epidemic; they also generated reports in other media as well as numerous invitations to the AIDS Task Force to speak at meetings.

The staff of Nashville CARES selected a modest goal; they did not want the local media to use the term "AIDS victims" because of its implication of passivity and stigma. So every time a reporter used that term, a staff member would write or call to complain. Slowly, the language began to change.

Jane Brody, health columnist for the *New York Times,* advised health educators to "find out who covers health-related stories and make your name and telephone number known to that person. Let them know what you are qualified to comment upon and that you are willing to be called and quoted."

Other observers suggest educating media personnel at a higher level. "There's a group of maybe a hundred people who produce 85 to 95 percent of all network drama; they can be reached and informed," noted George Gerbner of the University of Pennsylvania. If accurate messages on AIDS are included in soap operas, dramas, and situation comedies, millions of people can be educated. Gerbner suggested that professional organizations might be an appropriate vehicle for making contact with and educating producers.

Use all media, not just network television and daily newspapers, and use all possible avenues to get your messages into the media. AIDS educators have been creative in finding new ways to tap various media:

- The Cascade AIDS Project in Oregon sponsored a news conference for reporters from high school newspapers.
- Boston's AIDS Action Committee ran weekly advertisements explaining safer sex in a local gay newspaper.
- HERO worked with Baltimore's Black newspapers to provide accurate coverage of AIDS.
- GMHC produced a weekly show on AIDS for a local cable television network.

Thousands of small radio and television stations and newspapers reach millions of Americans. Getting coverage in the local weekly newspapers, the foreign-language radio station, or the late night call-in show can help reach targeted populations with specific messages. Getting coverage in the national media is difficult and time consuming. Most AIDS organizations would do well to focus on smaller outlets.

Having a news conference, demonstration, or clinic opening covered by the press is one way to make the news. But there are many other ways to get messages into the mass media: public service announcements (PSAs), letters to the editor, guest appearances on talk shows, and advertisements. Figure 15 lists different ways that AIDS educators can get their ideas into the mass media.

Do not assume that the media will cover your story as you present it. The primary goal of the media is not health education. "Both the print press and electronic outlets are private enterprises whose objective is to increase profits through increasing their audience," noted Harry Schwartz, a medical writer. "Sensationalism and exaggeration are time-tested means of gaining readers and viewers. AIDS was tailor-made for such treatment if only because Americans are so preoccupied about health."

"We have not found it hard to get the media to come to us," reported Lori Behrman, GMHC's media coordinator. "It has been harder to get the press to cover issues from our point of view. They shift focus from what GMHC thinks ought to be emphasized to what is coming out of the White House or what is being played up in the news at the time."

By understanding reporters' and editors' constraints, AIDS educators can plan media strategies more likely to meet their own goals as well as those of the media. For example, finding people with AIDS, IV drug users, or male prostitutes willing to discuss their experiences helps reporters give a human face to AIDS. Similarly, interviewing frontline workers about a program might make a better story than the executive director's perspective.

But educators also have to understand what the media cannot do. According to Laurie Garrett, a science reporter for National Public Radio, the media should not be the primary source of AIDS education. "It's not our job," she said, "and we aren't any good at it. We are not educators." Complicated messages, subtle distinctions, and sophisticated political analysis are unfortunately beyond the ability of most American mass media. Educators need to find other channels for this kind of communication.

Do not produce materials for the media without knowing that you can use them. The Seattle/Kings County Health Department's AIDS Project contracted with the Northwest AIDS Foundation to produce a PSA on AIDS. The spot featured two gay men discussing safer sex. After $10,000 was spent on the PSA, most local stations refused to run it. "The lesson we learned," said Ann Downer, an AIDS educator with the health department, "is never to produce anything without consulting with the media you want to carry the message." Images, words, and messages need to be discussed before money is spent. After this failure, the Northwest AIDS Foundation developed a strong relationship with the media, and radio and television producers are now coming to them to ask for guidance in producing stories. "In the future, said Downer, "we hope we don't need to spend money on this."

Integrate media appearances and media coverage of AIDS with other education strategies. While the Philadelphia AIDS Task Force was helping a reporter prepare the series of articles on AIDS in 1983, the group also developed a new brochure that it could send to people who would be requesting more information on AIDS after reading the articles.

Whenever a television show on AIDS is aired, the AIDS Project in Portland, Maine, brings in extra staff and volunteers to handle the increase in calls to the hotline.

Figure 15. HOW AIDS EDUCATORS CAN GET MEDIA COVERAGE

1. Hold a press conference to announce a program or event that your group is sponsoring.
2. Write a letter to the editor of your local daily or weekly newspaper.
3. Ask a well-known AIDS advocate to write an opinion editorial piece for the newspaper in your area.
4. Write a series of articles in your organization's newsletter about AIDS and what your group is doing to prevent AIDS. Include interesting photographs of your events. Ask other groups to reprint these articles in their newsletters.
5. Sponsor radio or television public service announcements (PSAs) about AIDS prevention or, more specifically, about the work your group is doing.
6. Suggest to a local cable television station that it host a show about AIDS prevention that features local prevention efforts.
7. Pay for (or co-sponsor with AIDS organizations) an AIDS prevention advertisement in the newspaper or on radio or television. Ask an advertising firm to donate its time and expertise to assist you.
8. Participate as a guest on a television or radio show about AIDS.
9. Insert safer-sex packets into newspapers. Include a condom if possible.
10. Involve celebrities in fund-raising activities, such as a benefit performance that would draw media attention. Or feature a famous person in an advertisement or PSA.
11. Involve community members in the development and evaluation of your media campaign.
12. Involve people with AIDS in radio or television talk shows about AIDS.
13. Organize a demonstration to support or oppose a media AIDS policy and invite reporters to attend.
14. Ask to meet with the editors of your local newspaper or television or radio station to discuss their AIDS coverage.
15. Send information on AIDS to regular columnists, asking them to write on a specific topic or your organization.
16. Offer to write a regular column on AIDS for your local newspaper, or host a regular program on AIDS on your local radio station.

HERO preceded its outreach program in Baltimore's Black community with briefings for journalists from the Black press. Their stories helped both to give HERO credibility and to disseminate accurate information.

These examples illustrate how AIDS organizations have used the media to strengthen or support other interventions. An effective strategy links program elements for reinforcement, publicity, and outreach.

Garry Anderson of the Portland AIDS Project stressed that he always asks reporters to publish or show the project's telephone number. "We have been very successful," he said, "in educating the media that they have the responsibility of giving resources to the public when they cover a story that is health related."

Media coverage of the AIDS epidemic has gone through several cycles of intense interest followed by relative neglect. AIDS organizations have often used the high points to good purpose. For many groups, the media's focus on Rock Hudson's illness provided the first opportunity to receive notice from reporters. Other organizations have used the media's "discovery" of AIDS among African-Americans and Latinos, adolescents, and IV drug users to get coverage of programs aimed at these populations. By carefully following, or even anticipating the media's perspective on AIDS, astute observers can seize the opportunity for timely access to listeners, viewers, and readers.

AIDS organizations should hire experts or develop their own expertise in media relations. Even for relatively small organizations, it probably makes sense to designate one person (or a small committee) as media coordinator. According to John Peterson, education director of the AIDS Project of the East Bay in Oakland, California, "If we had not had a media coordinator, we would simply not have been able to get the information out to meet the press's demands."

A media coordinator serves as liaison with reporters, arranges interviews, issues press releases, serves as spokesperson for the organization, and tracks media coverage. At best, the coordinator can establish personal relationships with local journalists, both answering questions and suggesting stories.

Larger organizations may want to hire media professionals to plan specific campaigns. The New York City Department of Health, for example, asked Saatchi and Saatchi Compton, one of the world's largest advertising agencies, to create a series of television and newspaper ads on AIDS. Taken on as a pro bono effort, the campaign targeted heterosexual women and stressed the use of condoms in preventing transmission of HIV infection. Although controversial, both the messages themselves and the media coverage of the campaign stimulated widespread discussion of AIDS. Similarly, the Illinois State Department of Health hired a major public relations firm to help develop its AIDS awareness campaign.

It would be a mistake, however, to turn over all responsibility for the media to advertising or public relations firms. Most of them lack expertise in the health field, and they are more used to selling products than informing people. AIDS educators should not be seduced by Madison Avenue glitz that looks attractive and professional but fails to communicate the desired message. By choosing goals *before* bringing in outside experts and by insisting on close collaboration throughout the process, AIDS organizations can increase the likelihood of effective campaigns.

Like other institutions in our society, the mass media are vulnerable to political pressure. Although newspapers and airwaves are owned by powerful individuals and corporations, AIDS organizations can work and have worked to change inadequate or inaccurate coverage. GMHC, for example, organized a demonstration at the *New York Times* to protest its failure to report on a huge benefit and received an unprecedented letter of apology from the editor. Subsequent coverage improved somewhat.

George Gerbner of the University of Pennsylvania suggested: "Health professionals and their organizations have the responsibility of making representations at license-renewal time to the Federal Communications Commission, of strengthening—instead of dismantling, as is now going on—the public protection, of broadening the sensitivities that are taken into account in the production of programs."

The success of AIDS organizations and public health professionals in overcoming opposition by at least some newspapers, magazines, and television stations to carrying either PSAs or advertisements for condoms attests to the possibility of overcoming the media's reluctance to become involved in controversial activities.

Training

AIDS educators provide training to give health workers and volunteers the knowledge and skills they need to take on specific responsibilities for the prevention of HIV infection. Training differs from more general AIDS education in that the primary goal is not to help individuals better protect themselves but rather to prepare staff or volunteers to add AIDS prevention to their work responsibilities. Figure 16 gives examples of how training has been used in AIDS education.

Benefits and Obstacles

What are the benefits of a training approach? First, training increases the pool of prevention workers. By helping teachers, nurses, social workers, prison guards, youth counselors, dormitory advisers, and others to educate their clients about AIDS, training disseminates the prevention message more widely throughout the population. An AIDS educator in a county health department spent all his time giving one-hour presentations in high schools throughout the county. A far more efficient use of his time would have been to train a few teachers in each school to take on this role.

Training is also a way of empowering other individuals, organizations, and communities. The older, larger AIDS organizations have sometimes been criticized for holding on to all the available resources. Training provides a vehicle for turning over expertise and skills to others who can use them. By sharing their experience with, for example, Black groups or agencies serving IV drug users, AIDS organizations can begin to address these groups' unequal access to resources. At the same time, new populations are being reached with AIDS prevention services.

Figure 16. EXAMPLES OF USES OF TRAINING IN AIDS PREVENTION PROGRAMS

Population To Be Trained	Skills To Be Developed
High school and college students	Educating peers about AIDS prevention.
Nurses and social workers	Counseling patients on AIDS risk reduction.
Beauty parlor operators	Providing customers with accurate information on AIDS.
Prostitutes or ex-prostitutes	Teaching safer sex to other prostitutes.
Physicians	Educating patients about AIDS.
Volunteers for telephone hotline	Answering callers' questions about AIDS.
Gay men	Leading safer-sex workshops for other gay men.
Counselors in drug treatment programs	Educating clients about AIDS prevention.

Finally, training uses existing resources, commitment, and motivation, freeing the educator from the necessity of starting from scratch. Teaching volunteers how to answer calls on a telephone hotline, drug counselors how to talk about safe sex, or teachers how to integrate AIDS into existing curricula builds on available skills, experience, and willingness to serve.

Trainers face a variety of obstacles, some specific to AIDS, others more general. Before an organization decides to provide training, it must identify a problem that can be addressed by this intervention. Because so many groups deny they have an AIDS problem, many never take the first step toward choosing to train their staff.

Another reason for reluctance to train is that it may require additional resources and release time for staff. For underfinanced, overburdened organizations, these two commodities can be difficult to negotiate.

Other organizations choose training inappropriately. A large hospital was mandated to offer AIDS testing and counseling to all patients. Rather than hire new staff, management chose to train nurses and social workers for this new task without diminishing their other responsibilities. Lack of resources, lack of clear policy guidelines, and uncertainty about institutional mission or priorities are unlikely to be solved by training. AIDS organizations can give training a bad name by using it for inappropriate purposes.

The views of an organization's administration on the purpose of training will strongly influence success. Training can be an attractive option for administrators unwilling to make a more costly, controversial, or appropriate choice. When training is offered to placate staff or clients or to give the appearance of action, it is unlikely to be effective.

Similarly, if trainees do not perceive a need for training, if they are not consulted about its content, or if they are forced to attend against their will, the likelihood of success is decreased. All these factors suggest that the political process of negotiating the training is as important as (and indeed inseparable from) the design of the curriculum.

Recommendations for Training

The following suggestions for developing effective training programs are aimed primarily at educators who work for voluntary or public AIDS organizations and who train both their own staff and volunteers in other organizations. A more detailed discussion on training of health workers can be found in Chapter 10.

Include trainees in planning the training. Research on training indicates that its effectiveness increases when trainees participate in choosing the goals, content, and methods. When trainees are already working in a setting, they understand the constraints and potentials of their situation better than anyone else. Only by meeting with drug counselor trainees before training started, for example, could trainers understand the depth of the trainees' feelings against teaching clients how to sterilize drug paraphernalia. If trainers decided to address this topic, they learned, they must discuss these feelings first.

According to Michael Carrera, a sex educator who trains health professionals in human sexuality, trainers must "take trainees where they are, not where you would like them to be." The only way of knowing the specific attitudes, feelings, and knowledge of a group is to communicate with them directly.

A variety of techniques are available for including trainees in the planning process. Ideally, the trainees establish a planning committee that includes trainees, trainers, and the management of the organization where the trainees work. This committee chooses goals, helps trainers decide on education strategies, and plans the evaluation. Faster and cheaper methods include meeting with a few trainees for discussions, surveying trainees, or (less desirable) asking for suggestions at the first session.

In some cases, management may resist giving trainees any role in the planning process. Trainers have an obligation to point out to the employer the potential costs of such a choice.

Include management in planning the training. Management support for training staff is essential. Penny Barchfeldt-Venet, director of AIDS education for the Philadelphia Department of Health, observed that "unless supervisors are committed to training, they can undo your work on staff education by creating fear and anxiety."

Management needs to assist in specifying the goals of training, identifying resources for it, providing release time for participants, and creating a supportive atmosphere. Most important, management can help ensure that trainees will have the opportunity to use the new knowledge and skills they acquire. Without this commitment, there is little point in carrying out a training program.

Sometimes, however, management itself needs help in understanding the issue. To address this issue, the AIDS Consortium of New York City ran a series of workshops for the boards and senior management of hospitals and health care institutions. Its goal was to help administrators understand the range of issues AIDS posed to the health care delivery system so that they could take action, including setting up in-service training programs to better prepare their agencies to cope with the epidemic. AIDS organizations can use the request for training as a starting point to help institutions define an agenda for action on AIDS.

Specify the objectives of the training program. Training programs require three levels of objectives. First, the planning team must identify those changes in service delivery that are expected to result from training. These improvements are presumed to contribute to improved health status for clients. Second, planners need to describe what new skills or behaviors trainees need in order to deliver the improved services. Finally, trainers must identify what trainees must learn in order to perform differently. Figure 17 illustrates objectives for a training program for AIDS counselors. Note that this process follows the health education planning model described in Chapter 3.

By carefully selecting specific objectives for a training program, planners make the purposes of the training clear to all involved parties. They also create a context for choosing education methods that will achieve their goals.

Evaluate the success of the training in achieving each level of objectives. Because training is designed to teach specific skills to a limited number of people, it is often easier to evaluate than general community education. And because many AIDS organizations conduct similar training programs repeatedly, the benefits of evaluation for improving the program are clear cut. The second column of Figure 17 suggests how trainers can evaluate changes in service delivery and the skills and knowledge of trainees. Chapter 3 provides more information on evaluation.

Set clear criteria for selecting trainees. Unlike community educators, who seek to reach as many people as possible, trainers need to select trainees who are likely to benefit from the program and use their new skills effectively. AIDS training programs attract recruits with a variety of motivations: desire to help people, personal

Figure 17. SAMPLE OUTCOMES FOR A FIVE-DAY PROGRAM FOR AIDS COUNSELORS*

	Desired Outcomes			
Changes in Service Delivery	Skills for Trainees	Knowledge for Trainees†	Possible Training Activities	How To Evaluate Success
Trainees will distribute condoms and demonstrate proper use at each clinic visit.	Ability to demonstrate condoms and instruct clients on use.	Proper condom use.	Presentation: "Talking With Your Clients About Sexuality" and "Name That Sex or Body Part" game.	Observation of participants during training activities.
	Ability to help clients eroticize safer sex and condom use.	Principles of safer sex (no exchange of body fluids).	Condom demonstration and role play.	Pretest and post-test training surveys of trainees' knowledge, attitudes, and behavior about safer sex and condom education.
	Ability to assist clients in talking to their partners about condoms.	Sensitivity to resistance to condoms that clients or their partners may exhibit.	Eroticizing safer-sex sex game: "Safer-Sex Continuum."	Comparison of condom distribution at clinic before and after training.
	Comfort discussing a range of sexual practices and life-styles with clients.	Awareness of a range of sexual behaviors and orientations.	"Working With a Resistant Condom User" exercise and discussion.	Observation of role play.
Trainees will provide AIDS risk reduction counseling at each clinic visit.	Ability to help clients assess their risk for HIV infection.	Knowledge of how HIV is transmitted and how to reduce risk of HIV infection.	Presentation: "What Your Clients Need To Know To Protect Themselves Against AIDS."	Pretraining and posttraining surveys of trainees' knowledge of AIDS prevention, and frequency and content of risk reduction counseling.
	Ability to assist clients in planning and carrying out a personal risk reduction strategy.	Knowledge of drug treatment referrals, hotlines, and other resources that would help clients reduce their risk.	Risk reduction counseling role plays.	Observation of participants during role plays.
	Ability to direct clients to services and resources that will assist risk reduction (drug treatment, condoms).	Knowledge of available resources and programs.	"AIDS Prevention Messages That You Can Give in 1 Minute, 5 Minutes, 15 Minutes. . ." Exercise.	Review of clients' charts for documentation of risk reduction counseling before and after training.

* See Figures 12 and 13 for other information on this training program.
† Trainees will be able to explain the following techniques, principles, and sensitivities.

concerns about AIDS, loneliness, or desire to change work responsibilities. What organization sponsors the training, whether it is voluntary or mandatory, and whether trainees will be paid for their work are among the questions that influence how trainees will be selected.

These are some of the selection procedures that AIDS organizations have used:

- Advertising the criteria for trainees (e.g., a desire to help people and at least one year of experience in counseling) and then letting trainees select themselves based on these criteria.
- Interviewing prospective trainees and rejecting those believed to be unsuitable.
- Inviting specific individuals to apply for or participate in training.
- Allowing anyone to participate in training, then testing participants to determine if they have learned desired skills. Only those who pass are "graduated."

Unless trainers develop methods to screen potential trainees, they may spend considerable time teaching people who will never use the training presented. Whichever option or combination is selected, trainers can avoid creating resentment and hurt feelings and providing inadequate services by specifying selection criteria at the outset.

Address cognitive, affective, and behavioral dimensions of trainees' understanding of AIDS. Dennis James, health care provider educator for Boston's AIDS Action Committee, reported that his training sessions "go straight to emotions." Otherwise, he observed, "all the facts in the world cannot break through the fears, denial, and anxiety people feel about AIDS." Too often, educators see training as a straightforward recital of information or demonstration of skills. They assume, often falsely, that trainees are not infected by the epidemic of fear that has accompanied AIDS. The AIDS Action Committee, like many other groups, has found that educators who have AIDS themselves are particularly effective at unfreezing people's stereotypes and anxieties.

At the same time, trainers need to distinguish between affective issues that influence a trainee's work and those that are primarily personal. The former are appropriate for discussion in the training session; the latter are usually not. Drawing the dividing line is not always easy. In a program for drug counselors, for example, many of whom were former addicts, information on risk factors for HIV infection had intensely personal meaning as well as professional impact. Trainers emphasized that the sessions they presented were intended to help counselors understand their own feelings as they affected job performance. Judy Macks of the San Franciso AIDS Health Project suggested that by "letting it be known that your organization is available to help," trainers can reassure individuals who need services beyond the training sessions.

Bringing to the surface trainees' feelings about sexuality, drugs, death, and their clients can precipitate an emotional crisis. "Working in the affective domain," said sex educator Carrera, "can lead to unzipping feelings, and trainers have to know how to zip, to help people get their feelings back together."

Choosing experienced and well-educated trainers minimizes such problems, as does careful planning. By specifying what trainees are expected to be able to do at the end of the process, trainers have a simplistic but clear criterion for including or excluding a particular topic. If it helps achieve the goal, it is worth considering. If it does not, then it is inappropriate.

Provide trainees with ongoing support, feedback, and supervision. By extending a training program over a longer period (e.g., four two-hour sessions for four weeks rather than one day), it is possible for trainees to practice new skills. Each session can begin with a report on this practice, and trainers can critique the performance.

Trainers have a responsibility to make sure that trainees can use the skills they learn. This can be accomplished by meeting with trainees several weeks or months after the program to discuss problems. Establishing ongoing support groups of trainees or periodic refresher sessions can also achieve this end. Still another possibility is to provide more extensive training to some staff or supervisors to enable them to provide further supervision. Finally, letting trainees know about other education programs allows them to continue learning.

Use training to achieve other organizational goals. Nashville CARES offered a training program for health and social service workers that yielded new contacts in agencies providing services for people with AIDS.

By providing sessions for teachers on AIDS, the Philadelphia Department of Health established a rapport with the school system before the issue of admitting children with AIDS arose.

GMHC uses its training programs to publicize its hotline, find new outlets for distributing its literature, and make contact with new organizations.

By integrating various program elements, AIDS organizations can increase their impact on the populations they serve. Training can be an important outreach activity that helps organizations to reach new populations, recruit new volunteers and staff, and develop new coalitions and networks. By considering these less obvious outcomes of training, educators can design programs so that these benefits are realized as fully as possible.

Condom Campaigns

Increasing the number of people who use condoms during sexual activity that involves the exchange of semen, blood, or vaginal secretions has been a major goal of AIDS educators. For some, it is the primary mission. "If we can get every gay man in Boston to wear a condom every time he has sex," said one educator working for the AIDS Action Council, "we'd have won half the battle against AIDS."

Typical Goals of Condom Campaigns

Using all the education strategies described in previous sections, AIDS organizations have launched condom campaigns to achieve the following goals:

- make people aware of the condom's benefits in preventing AIDS, other STDs, and unwanted pregnancies;
- increase the availability of condoms;
- increase the acceptability of their use;
- teach people how to use condoms correctly;
- help people negotiate the use of condoms with their sexual partners.

A variety of activities have been used to achieve these objectives. In San Francisco, Los Angeles, New York City, and other places, health departments or AIDS organizations have sponsored PSAs on television, radio, and in the newspapers promoting condom use to prevent AIDS.

Throughout the country, AIDS groups have distributed free condoms at health clinics, gay bars, colleges, health fairs, and other events. The New York City Health Department has trained more than 120 of its employees to counsel and educate clients about condom use. Universities, bars, and other organizations have installed condom-dispensing machines in places accessible to patrons. Health officials have urged pharmacists to play an active role in displaying condoms and making their purchase easier. Other ideas for promoting condom use are listed in Figure 18.

Common Fallacies About Condoms

Planners of condom campaigns report that they frequently encounter attitudes and beliefs among health professionals working on this issue that can block effective programs. Among them are the following.

"Condoms are easy to use; therefore it is sufficient simply to demonstrate their use." In fact, complex cultural, emotional, sexual, and gender role factors influence condom use. Educators need to learn how these factors interact among the specific individuals and groups they serve. Moreover, many people do not know how to use condoms properly. Demonstrations should include practice sessions using models and an opportunity for questions and answers.

"Women are the appropriate target for condom campaigns." Correctly noting that women have traditionally been responsible for contraception, that they are more likely to practice preventive health behaviors, and that they now buy more than 40% of the condoms sold in the United States, health workers have assumed that women are more likely than men to be persuaded about the benefits of condom use.

Although this assumption may be correct, it ignores the fact that ultimately it is men who must decide whether to use condoms. More important, targeting condom campaigns at women accepts the notion that women *should* be solely responsible for health. Not only does this place an unfair burden on women, it also undercuts a central theme of AIDS education: that *everyone* needs to take action to prevent AIDS.

"Women have enough power in their relationships to negotiate with partners about condom use." Condom campaigns that seek only to make condoms available, increase knowledge about their correct use, and motivate people to use them will not help the woman who wants to use condoms but has a partner who refuses. Effective education must help women develop strategies that both acknowledge and challenge male resistance to condom use. It must also help men to reexamine their negative attitudes.

A variant of this assumption is that women, especially African-American and Latina women, have no control in their relationships and that therefore discussing condoms is useless. Such pessimistic assumptions undercut effective interventions.

"Campaigns should not address the contraceptive benefits of condoms." Several factors discourage AIDS educators from discussing condoms as a method of birth control: opposition from religious groups, parents, and some elected officials; gay organizations' desire to emphasize the role of condoms in preventing disease to make them more acceptable to gay men; health workers' reluctance to generate more controversy about AIDS, especially on an issue perceived to be extraneous; and the family planning establishment's hesitation about condoms as an effective method of birth control.

On the other hand, for many heterosexual couples and especially teenagers, the prevention of pregnancy can be as urgent a life task as the prevention of AIDS. By refusing to address this need, AIDS organizations miss an opportunity to develop a more comprehensive approach to health. Given the related epidemics of

Figure 18. METHODS OF PROMOTING CONDOMS

- Contact pharmacists and their professional associations and other retail stores to make sure that condoms and spermicides are displayed in the open. AIDS information should also be available to customers.
- Hold special events that involve condom distribution, such as Valentine's Day, Halloween condom costume contests, Fathers' and Mothers' Days.
- Develop creative or amusing ways to package condoms to appeal to a variety of consumers—for example, in fortune cookies or in special carrying cases.
- Include condoms in safer-sex information packets given to clients in family planning and health clinics.
- Contact local sex shops to give out free condoms to customers.
- Contact video stores to include condoms with rentals of erotic films.
- Contact makers of erotic films to encourage them to make safer-sex films, to have safer-sex demonstrations as previews to films, or to show condom use in films.
- Develop PSAs that encourage condom use and give information on where to get them free.
- Organize campaigns to encourage media to use such PSAs.
- Use television, magazine, and billboard advertisements for condoms.
- Write to television networks and print media to encourage them to advertise condoms.
- Solicit celebrities and local leaders to back your campaign publicly.
- Involve community groups in promoting condoms. Sponsor joint events at which condoms can be distributed, such as health fairs, or "condo" dances in which a condom is the entry ticket.
- Install condom dispensers in male and female public bathrooms. College dorms, bars, discos, health clubs, and movie theaters are good places to start.
- Write letters to the editor of local newspapers, community newsletters, or organizations' bulletins about your condom campaign. Encourage reporters and editors to write stories.
- Encourage condom companies to develop new strategies for marketing using nonprofit or community groups.
- Sponsor condom comfort workshops to help people overcome obstacles to using them.
- Train health workers to discuss condoms comfortably with their clients and to help clients solve problems.
- Distribute condoms at all AIDS education events.
- Encourage drug programs, prisons, runaway shelters, and other institutions that serve people at risk of AIDS to distribute condoms.

syphilis, gonorrhea, and other STDs, HIV infection, and teenage pregnancy, the failure to emphasize both functions of condoms has contributed to a public health crisis.

For some feminists, the refusal to discuss condoms as contraceptives suggests the old sexual double standard: Men deserve to have information on how to protect themselves and their partners against disease so they can enjoy sex more fully; women, however, are not entitled to information on how to prevent an unwanted pregnancy.

"Public opposition to more open discussion of condoms is so great that condom campaigns should not be a high priority." The opposition of religious and conservative political groups to condom advertising and distribution has led some health officials and AIDS organizations to shy away from this activity. However, a 1987 poll conducted by Louis Harris for Planned Parenthood Federation of America found that 60% of American adults believed that television stations should carry condom advertisements. When reminded that Surgeon General Koop and the National Academy of Sciences have called for increased use of condoms to prevent the spread of AIDS, the percentage of those favoring television condom ads rose to 74%.

Moreover, a 1987 random survey of more than 600 television and radio stations found that 20% already accepted condom advertisements and 67% of the television stations say they will do so in the future. By bowing to conservative pressure, public health officials miss an opportunity to provide leadership.

"Condoms are the solution to the prevention of AIDS." Using condoms is one of the most concrete, positive steps that AIDS educators can offer. It allows people to continue sexual activity with some significant protection against a lethal disease. For these reasons, it is easy for educators to promote condom use uncritically. Several factors argue against this strategy.

First, although most experts agree that condoms provide important protection against HIV infection, they do not provide total safety. Studies of contraceptive effectiveness show that condoms fail to prevent pregnancy for at least one couple out of ten who rely on the method for a year. Many studies show even higher failure rates. It is likely that HIV transmission occurs more readily than conception. In 1987, the Food and Drug Administration required the leading manufacturers to recall 100,000 condoms after a spot check showed that an excessive number of them leaked. Other researchers belive that condoms are more likely to rip or pull off during anal intercourse than vaginal intercourse. Thus, responsible AIDS educators must find ways to talk about condoms positively and accurately, without giving learners a false sense of security.

Uncritical promotion of condoms is also unlikely to be effective. Powerful religious, sexual, and cultural factors block the use of condoms. Unless these deeply rooted attitudes are addressed, people's behavior is unlikely to change. Most condom campaigns have not by themselves been sufficiently intense to overcome these obstacles.

Finally, distribution of condoms does not guarantee their use. Unless men and women are willing to use condoms and spermicides every time they have sexual intercourse, the protection provided is limited. Unfortunately, there is no quick fix for AIDS prevention. Changing sexual behavior requires a variety of interventions over an extended time.

Community Education

As the AIDS epidemic spreads beyond gay and bisexual men and IV drug users, AIDS educators need to find new ways to reach ever broader sectors of the population. Given that AIDS is a social and political problem as well as a medical one, every person in the United States needs to understand the dimensions of the AIDS epidemic and contribute to finding solutions. Still another reason for broad-based public education is that programs aimed at gay men or IV drug users will not reach all those at risk of sexual or drug-related transmission of HIV infection. All these reasons combine to make community AIDS education an attractive strategy for reaching those in need of information or skills.

Many activities fall under the rubric of community education, but in this discussion it will be defined narrowly. Community AIDS education refers to those activities designed to prevent the spread of HIV infection undertaken by community-based organizations (CBOs) not primarily focused on AIDS.

Social scientists have long struggled to define "community." Here, "community" describes a population living in a specific physical environment and sharing certain values, institutions, and leadership. Note that it is *not* assumed that communities are homogeneous culturally, ethnically, or economically. Note also that this definition excludes concepts such as the gay community or the Latino community that lack a geographic focus. That formulation will be considered in Section II. Certainly, ethnic, national, and sexual identity play a key role in targeting AIDS education. Too often, however, AIDS educators have overlooked the equally useful forum that geographic communities provide.

The term CBO, often used to refer to any group located in a community setting, also requires definition. Here, three specific characteristics distinguish CBOs from other institutions. First, CBOs have a defined geographic "catchment" area. Second, they have a mission that relates to the community as a whole, not only to individuals in the community. Third, community residents participate in making organizational decisions.

These criteria do not necessarily provide a clear-cut "yes" or "no" answer to the question "Is this group a CBO?" Rather, they help define a continuum on which community workers can locate specific groups. A welfare office located in a particular community would not meet these criteria, nor would the branch office of a citywide or national centralized organization. Large regional AIDS organizations do not meet this definition either, because they usually interact with many geographic communities. A neighborhood association, however, or a group working to improve local schools would fit this definition.

CBOs offer AIDS educators a variety of advantages. First, they have a defined constituency and an organizational structure; educators don't need to pursue the time-consuming tasks of seeking an audience and developing a group. Second, these organizations have credibility among their constituents; educators can "borrow" the trust inherent in such relationships. Third, these groups have often defined a mission that corresponds to the perceived needs of some community residents. By looking for ways to integrate AIDS prevention into this existing mission, educators can increase the likelihood that they and their clients share certain goals. Finally, CBOs often have intimate and detailed understanding of their constituents, which, if conveyed accurately to educators, can increase the likelihood of effective communication. For all these reason, CBOs also provide AIDS educators with clear-cut economic benefits, because several steps of the planning process may already have occurred.

Few CBOs will be able to hire a specialized AIDS educator, but many groups have resources and expertise that can be used for AIDS education. How then can AIDS educators help CBOs take on AIDS prevention activities? Among the services AIDS organizations have provided are—

- developing specialized written materials such as AIDS brochures to be used by adult literacy or English-as-a-second-language programs;
- offering training programs for community leaders to help them understand and act on AIDS;
- providing a series of workshops on AIDS for the youth program in a housing project's tenants council;
- training ministers and other church leaders to provide AIDS prevention counseling;
- helping the staff of a neighborhood health center to provide their patients with risk reduction education.

Each of these activities requires defining the intersection between the missions of the AIDS organization and of the CBO. The extent to which both groups perceive the effort to be important will determine the success of the collaborative effort. When staff of AIDS organizations assume that the CBO staff will share their priority for AIDS prevention, problems can ensue.

Obstacles to Community Education

Wherever AIDS educators turn, they encounter denial that AIDS is a problem, and CBOs are no exception. Groups that do not work directly with people who have AIDS are particularly likely to think it is not their problem. For example, Rashidah Hassan of Blacks Educating Blacks About Sexual Health Issues (BEBASHI) reported that at first Black ministers in Philadelphia were reluctant to discuss AIDS because they feared their parishioners didn't want to hear about it in church. Once they saw that members of their congregation were dying of AIDS, they were more willing to speak out.

Another reason why CBOs hesitate to take on the AIDS issue is a fear of being stigmatized. The staff of a neighborhood health center in the Bronx, New York, for example, were reluctant to accept a special AIDS program because they were afraid their patients would stay away from a facility identified as an AIDS center that served drug addicts. This health clinic had worked hard to attract working families to their facility and did not want to risk losing what they had achieved.

Other CBOs do not want to address an issue perceived to be identified with gay men. Clients too can be affected by the stigmatization of AIDS. According to Judy Wenning of the West Side AIDS Project, a New York City program sponsored by a settlement house, some people are less willing to use an AIDS service in a community organization where people might know them.

Most CBOs already feel overburdened: too much to do, too few resources, too many problems in their community. These groups feel overwhelmed when they are asked to add AIDS to their mission, especially given the negative social attitudes toward the disease. Unless AIDS educators can present the request for added activities in a way that makes sense to the group, it is unlikely that the group will agree or, if they do agree, that they will provide adequate services. Figure 19 suggests how AIDS prevention can be defined to be relevant to various community groups.

Recommendations for Community Education

The following recommendations are aimed at AIDS educators working for state

Figure 19. COMMUNITY ORGANIZATIONS CAN PLAY A ROLE IN AIDS PREVENTION

Organization	How Group Might Define Problem	Activities
Neighborhood or block association	Concern for general welfare of residents; need for additional community resources.	Community forum; health fair; distribute pamphlets around the neighborhood and at meetings.
Church or synagogue	Concern for spiritual and physical health of parishioners.	Pastoral counseling; sermons on AIDS; education programs; training of volunteer educator advocacy; article in parish bulletin.
Neighborhood health center	As component of primary and preventive care.	Patient counseling; community education; speakers' bureau; condom distribution.
Parents' association	Need to protect well-being of children now and in future.	Education for children; parent education; distribution of education materials.
Child care center	Need to protect well-being of children now and in future; need to protect staff.	Parent and staff education; basic health education for children; distribution of education materials.
Youth or recreation program	Provide young people with knowledge and skills to protect themselves.	Training peer counselors; education programs; distribution of materials; condom distribution.
Civic group (Lions, Elks, Kiwanis, Junior League)	Concern for community welfare.	Fundraising; community forums; lobbying and advocacy; education.
Chamber of Commerce	Social problem leading to lost production or social and community division.	Funding; political support; or consciousness raising among business leaders; assisting and consulting on instituting education in workplace; helping businesses develop policies.
Community newspaper	Human interest; medical news; threat to community health; political response to epidemic.	Scientific news articles; editorials; columns' coverage of community forums; interviews with AIDS educators and advocates.
Political group	Opportunity to organize community people to mobilize resources.	Advocacy; education; legislative work.
Settlement house	Community welfare, particularly for low-income groups.	Training; education programs; peer counselors; advocacy.
Social club	Concern for community welfare; concern for their members.	Building awareness among the membership and in the community; sponsoring forums, poster contests; consulting on development of education materials.
Library	Community education.	Resource file on AIDS; meeting space; distribution of pamphlets, film festivals.
Literacy, high school equivalency, or English-as-a-second-language program	Vehicle for teaching academic and social skills.	Development of special teaching materials; distribution of pamphlets.

or local health departments, designated AIDS organizations, and other large voluntary groups. They are designed to help these workers assist CBOs with integrating AIDS prevention into their activities. As more resources for AIDS eduction become available, some larger CBOs may hire their own educators, who can also use these suggestions.

Use requests for information on AIDS to establish a relationship with CBOs. Jim Holmes, director of the GMHC Speakers Bureau, explained: "A few years ago when a community group called to ask for a speaker we sent someone out, that person gave a talk, and that was it. Now we try to be more sophisticated. I will meet with the group and ask them what they hope to accomplish. We'll sit down and discuss what GMHC can do and what their group can do. When the speaker leaves, we have started a process, not ended it."

Most AIDS organizations provide a variety of services to the community as a whole—speakers, brochures, and films. This is an important function that will continue to be needed. By using every request for such services as an opportunity to discuss how the requesting organization can take on a piece of AIDS prevention, designated AIDS groups can multiply their impact.

AIDS organizations need not wait for CBOs to come to them. If a group wants to reach Blacks or Latinos, youth, or women, it can initiate contact with CBOs working with these constituencies. By offering to provide services, the AIDS group can establish a relationship with an organization that can help both groups achieve their goals.

Negotiate a realistic set of goals that both the AIDS organization and the CBO feel comfortable with. The preliminary discussions that define the contract between two groups shape the climate in which the relationship develops. AIDS educators need to listen to what the CBO wants. If they assume they know everything they need to know about how to plan a program, they are unlikely to be trusted by CBO staff or to meet perceived needs.

At the same time, AIDS organizations need to set limits on what they can and cannot do. As Judy Spiegel of AIDS Project Los Angeles explained, "Most agencies don't want to acknowledge their limitations." As a result, she said, promises that cannot be fulfilled are made and bad feelings result.

The goal of negotiations is to agree on a plan for shared activities, not to agree on everything about AIDS. Thus, groups like Nashville CARES and Boston's AIDS Action Committee consented to help conservative church groups plan education programs even though they differed in their views on homosexuality. "Our goal," said AIDS Action Committee's Bryanne Camella, "was to make sure that accurate information gets out. Later, we can discuss our political differences."

By engaging CBO staff in a dialogue, AIDS educators create the opportunity for an ongoing relationship. Moreover, research in organizational development strongly confirms the view that a mutually defined agenda is more likely to maintain support than a unilateral one.

Look for ways to transfer the AIDS organization's knowledge, skills, and experience to the CBO. Providing a service and moving on meets an immediate need, but empowering a group to meet future needs on its own ensures lasting benefits. This second goal requires a different style of work. "We're making a lot more collaborative efforts and not just trying to do it all on our own," said Judy Spiegel of AIDS Project Los Angeles. "We're trying to build from the ground up."

Specific activities that transfer expertise to staff of CBOs include training, leadership development, shared planning and evaluation, and joint efforts to find resources.

Once a relationship has developed, find ways for CBOs to help achieve other goals of the AIDS organization. To establish a successful relationship, the first priority of AIDS organizations is to help the CBO achieve its goals. Once that end has been achieved, broader collaborative efforts can be started.

AIDS organizations can use CBOs to publicize services such as hotlines, support groups, and speakers bureaus. CBOs can distribute educational materials, condoms, or bleach to clean needles. CBOs can also join political coalitions to advocate for prevention policies or more resources for AIDS prevention.

Enlist people with AIDS to help plan and deliver community education. "One of the biggest problems we're having," said Mark Friedman of the Pittsburgh AIDS Task Force, "is that since there are so few cases in Pittsburgh, people don't feel vulnerable. One way to get at this is to have people with AIDS do public education."

Giving AIDS a human face, report educators from around the country, is a vital step in public education. First, it makes the threat more real, more concrete, thus motivating risk reduction behavior. Second, it helps to reduce anxiety and discrimination and to increase empathy. Meeting a person with AIDS who looks not so different from us, who describes the day-to-day problems of the disease, who struggles to maintain dignity in this experience, helps to create the human bonds that blunt prejudice and fear. Third, for many people with AIDS, public education provides an important way to give their experience meaning and to contribute to the fight to control AIDS. Many AIDS organizations have developed respectful and effective way to engage people with AIDS in their education, and CBOs can benefit from their experiences.

Define the goals for joint efforts in a way that will help the CBO fulfill its existing mission. Few groups will be willing to drop their existing activities to take on AIDS, but because AIDS is linked with so many other issues, it is often possible to find common areas of interest. Groups seeking to lower rates of teenage pregnancy, for example, need to talk about contraception and relationships, which provides an opportunity for discussing AIDS prevention. Neighborhood groups addressing drug abuse problems can easily add AIDS to their rationale for action.

Linking AIDS goals to other existing goals can also strengthen a group's self-confidence by emphasizing its existing expertise on the subject. This counteracts the tendency to see AIDS as an overwhelming and totally new problem.

Politically, strengthening a group's understanding of and commitment to AIDS prevention lays the groundwork for building the coalitions and networks that were described in Chapter 2.

S E C T I O N   T W O

Reaching Out: How To Educate Specific Population Groups About AIDS

For the first years of the epidemic, AIDS educators worked primarily in the gay community and with IV drug users. But as the epidemic spreads, education needs to reach new groups who are at risk for AIDS.

The recognition that it was specific behaviors that led to HIV infection—sexual encounters in which partners exchanged body fluids and the sharing of virus-contaminated needles and drug works—rather than sexual preference or drug addiction per se influenced AIDS educators to focus on those behaviors rather than on a group identity. This new insight helped mitigate the stigmatization that early forms of AIDS education seemed to encourage. "It's not who you are," said AIDS educators, "it's what you do that puts you at risk."

But as with other forms of education, effective AIDS educators must acknowledge that each community, each population group, has its own values, norms, culture, and networks of communication. Thus, most AIDS education has been targeted at a specific sector of the population. The following chapters describe the experiences and problems of AIDS educators working with gay and bisexual men, IV drug users, African-Americans and Latinos, youth, women, workers, prisoners, people with hemophilia, homeless people, and people with developmental disabilities. Several chapters begin with brief case histories describing specific projects.

The goal of this section is to help educators working with specific populations to develop appropriate education interventions that reflect some of the lessons learned in the first eight years of the epidemic.

CHAPTER FIVE

Gay and Bisexual Men

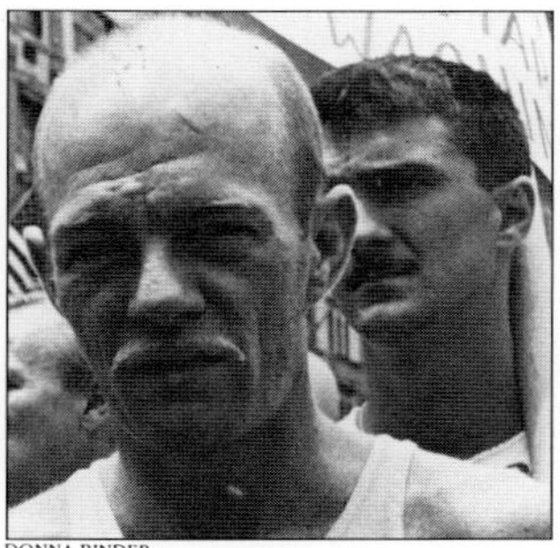
DONNA BINDER

CASE HISTORY

Educating Gay and Bisexual Men in Utah About AIDS

More than 65% of Utah's 1.6 million residents are Mormons. The political, social, and cultural climates of the state are strongly influenced by the Mormon religion, which condemns sexual activity outside marriage, sex education, drug use, and homosexuality. This climate creates unique challenges for AIDS educators.

Because of these conservative values, many in Utah did not expect AIDS would ever become a problem in their state. But by the beginning of 1988, there were 113 reported cases of AIDS in Utah, and since 1983, 72 persons with AIDS have died. As in the rest of the country, the number of reported cases in Utah is doubling each year. An AIDS researcher in Salt Lake City likens it to being "run over by a slow freight train."

Since Utah is so dominated by a religion that equates homosexuality with murder, heresy, and adultery, many gay men are forced into bisexuality. Mormon leaders attempt to "cure" homosexuality by encouraging gay men to marry women. But now, in the face of the AIDS epidemic, even the Mormon leadership realizes that this "cure" is not only ineffective, it is also dangerous. Many gay men in Utah, both Mormon and non-Mormon, marry or date women because of this intense social and religious pressure and then, as one gay man put it, "play around on the side, dropping their dates off at 10 and then going to a gay bar."

State health officials call married gay men "a cause for great concern," fearing that they will infect their wives and future children. Craig Nichols, the state epidemiologist, estimates that there are 30,000 homosexual and bisexual men in Utah, a number that gay community leaders assert is a significant underestimate. They describe Salt Lake City as an immigrant city—as one said, "the only big city in the middle of nowhere. Plus it has a well-publicized gay community. It's a magnet for gay people in the region."

Both public health officials and gay community leaders agree that most homosexual men in Utah are not openly gay. The implications of this for effective AIDS education for gay and bisexual men is the subject of rancorous disputes between public health officials and the gay community. In Utah, five years after the first reported case of AIDS, the issue of who is responsible for providing education for men at highest risk for AIDS has yet to be resolved.

Where AIDS is concerned, Utah's public health officials feel that they are walking on a perilous tightrope, balancing the demands of the gay community against what they see as the limits imposed by the political leadership. Jessalyn Pittman, director of Utah's AIDS Control Program, explained: "Utah is a very conservative state. I know that taxpayers' money will not ever be used to dispense condoms. We can talk about them, but we can't push them. During our presentations we use CDC [Centers for Disease Control] slides that say 'Use condoms.' We can't demonstrate how to use condoms, either. We tell our audiences to read the instructions on the box."

Moreover, Nichols (the state epidemiologist) believed that any explicit discussions of safer sex were also impermissible. "I don't think that the state has the responsibility to teach proper condom usage," he said. "We'll do the things we know we can do and that are acceptable and other groups will have to fill in where they think there is a deficit. Any explicit discussion of the risks of gay sex must come from the gay community itself."

Leaders of the gay community have expressed outrage at the state health department's attitude. Graham Bell, a member of People Concerned About AIDS (PCAA), said: "We have been trying to work with state and county health officials since 1985. We went to them repeatedly to discuss the situation. The state health department said it was the county's responsibility. The county said they didn't have any funds, that the state controlled all the money for AIDS. They all just passed the buck."

Patty Reagan, a founder of the Salt Lake City AIDS Foundation, added, "The state hasn't had one public health program for gay people. They had all these programs for doctors, nurses, and the Junior League. They've done it for everybody but the gay community."

Nichols denied these charges. He and his staff maintained that "the gay community in Salt Lake City is a small, vocal minority of the homosexuals in Utah." In a proposal submitted to the CDC, the state contended that "health education and risk reduction services are provided to gay and bisexual men primarily through counseling which occurs before and after HIV testing," and that "the only way to reach closeted gays is through mass media. Thus, efforts to educate the general public will have the additional benefit of addressing the educational needs of gay and bisexual men." Bell and other members of the gay community suggested that distributing literature and condoms at gay bars and doing education programs at the 26 gay organizations around the state might have been more effective.

Bell formed PCAA to mobilize the gay community's anger about the state's lack of responsiveness into action. The group's first act was to publicly call for Nichols' resignation because of alleged "dereliction of duty" evidenced by not educating high-risk groups about AIDS. PCAA called press conferences and circulated petitions because, according to Bell, "Although the gay community was angry about the state's lack of action, it was still hard to get people to put their name or face on the line." These actions attracted significant media attention.

Other AIDS organizations and gay leaders disagreed with Bell's and PCAA's angry, confrontational tactics. Bell's response was, "If you have no power, what are you left with? In my opinion, the state doesn't care about us. If moral appeals don't work, what are you left with except confrontation?" In Bell's opinion, some of the other AIDS organizations were worried about "biting the hand that feeds them. But the problem was that they weren't getting fed! The state was openly hostile to them. They [state officials] would talk to them, but not give them any money or help."

Pittman of the AIDS Control Program denied that the gay community's needs had been ignored by the state's AIDS programs. According to Pittman, "They haven't asked us for help, only for funds. The gay community is doing a good job of educating itself." But now that funds are available, she admitted that "there's a political problem with funding gay organizations. We can find an AIDS-oriented group, but not if they promote gay rights or gay sex. This is a very conservative state. In no way do taxpayers want their money used to promote homosexuality."

CASE HISTORY

Gay Men's Health Crisis, New York City

Five years ago today, a group of men came together and founded GMHC. Since that time, over 3,000 dedicated men and women have walked through our doors. Let us all go forward with renewed hope and spirit.

This proclamation was made to several hundred of those volunteers gathered at a reception in February 1987, to celebrate the fifth anniversary of Gay Men's Health Crisis (GMHC). In those five years of existence, GMHC had grown from a group of friends who raised $769.55 one weekend by collecting money outside a gay disco to an "AIDS Service and Education Foundation" with more than 60 full-time employees, more than 1,000 active volunteers, a mortgage on a new building, and an operating budget of $3.5 million.

GMHC's story actually began in July 1981 when the *New York Times* printed an article announcing a "Rare Cancer in 41 Homosexuals." The following month writer Larry Kramer called together a group of friends to see what action could be taken. More than 80 men gathered in Kramer's apartment. The doctor who had made the *New York Times* announcement told this group that the reported cases represented just the tip of the iceberg, that things were going to get much worse. His suggestion was to organize to inform the community of the danger and to raise money for research, which he projected would be difficult, since the disease had occurred mainly in gay men. By December of that year these men had raised $11,806.55 to contribute to New York University Medical Center's Kaposi's Sarcoma Fund.

In January 1982, GMHC got its name when one of the founding members sighed, "Gay men certainly have a health crisis." At that time it was still accepted, even among the gay community, that AIDS was a gay disease. That perception did not change until months later when the disease began to be referred to as acquired immune deficiency syndrome.

Recognition of the problem in the gay community was also slow. GMHC's first official fundraiser, "Showers," held in April 1982, got such poor advance support that it was decided to disband the organization if the event was not a success. The $32,086 netted, however, assured GMHC's future, and plans were made to incorporate.

The earliest organized service of GMHC was its AIDS hotline, started in May 1982 and staffed entirely by volunteers. Today that hotline fields between 4,000 and 5,000 calls per month, educating callers about AIDS and making referrals to services provided by GMHC and others.

At the same time the client services program began, sending volunteers into hospitals to visit people with AIDS. This identified another early education need. Diego Lopez, GMHC's second clinical director, started professional education by going into the hospitals to teach their staffs how to care for people with AIDS.

Soon GMHC's first public AIDS forum was held in New York City and 500 people attended. In June 1982, GMHC's first newsletter was published; 50,000 copies were printed and shipped all over the world. GMHC's first office space was acquired in September 1982 and the following month, GMHC assisted in setting up AIDS Atlanta. Hence, as early as 1982 GMHC became a resource for other AIDS organizations in their early stages, an education function that continues and grows today.

On November 19, 1982, Larry Kramer, Dr. Dan William, and Phil Lanzaratta represented GMHC on the "Phil Donahue Show," the first national television AIDS show. Such public appearances remain one of the most broad-reaching education functions of GMHC.

In November and December 1982, 250,000 copies of GMHC's health recommendations brochure were distributed in bars all over New York City. GMHC's first set of safer-sex guidelines was funded by the New York City Department of Health and the New York City Police Department. The issues had become of enough concern that public funding had begun to trickle in.

Today at any one time GMHC is providing services to more than 1,000 people with AIDS and their families and friends. In addition, it provides advocacy for all of these people and for other people at risk, as well as education to all segments of the population. What are some of the issues GMHC faces concerning education? Where are these issues taking GMHC?

Dr. Charles McKinney, director of education of GMHC, said the agency is now in the process of "professionalizing." He pointed out that GMHC came together in response to needs that were not being met by other social institutions. The people who developed GMHC's early programs were not necessarily trained to develop those programs, but GMHC was able to respond more quickly and perhaps better than other social institutions, because GMHC was not held back by professional disciplines. "Because 'can't' wasn't an option," McKinney said, "we got the job done."

"Professionalizing," however, is a delicate task, McKinney explained, because *people with professional credentials are responsible for developing those same social institutions which were unable to respond to the crisis. It was people who were not limited and held back by the disciplines of their professions who responded. While we don't want people who are not trained as social workers and psychologists behaving as social workers and psychologists, we don't want the type of trained people in here that are going to transform GMHC into the same type of social institution outside that has been absolutely unresponsive and who are looking to us as the model of what social service agencies ought to be.*

The vitality of GMHC's education programs, McKinney believed, stems from the materials that the education department has developed to fit its curriculum. Because no materials existed and financial resources to develop new ones were limited, the education programs had to be innovative. "Our model was developed to address the needs which were identified, and so flexibility and immediacy of response were parts of the model," he stated. "We were not shackled with a predisposed model."

To this end, McKinney said, it is important to "keep this department from being cluttered with the restraints that are built into the skills that educators use." He cited as an example the AIDS prevention program that GMHC took into the bars and the bathhouses. GMHC presented the program to the audience at 4:00 AM on Sunday, a time that was convenient for the learners, not the educators.

GMHC's experience in educating gay men prompted the New York City Department of Health to fund some of its education programs. As a volunteer organization, GMHC has used language and visuals that offend some segments of society but that, it has been proven, are the most effective means of educating gay men. Because the Health Department is a public agency, it may fall under attack for using such education materials, making GMHC a viable route for reaching gay men.

Just whom the agency is going to serve has surfaced as a controversial issue. Larry Kramer, in an open letter to GMHC published in the *New York Native* on January 26, 1987, criticized GMHC for attempting "to be all things for all people, in doing so losing complete sight of what you should be doing and not doing." He was particularly critical of GMHC's alleged failure to play a more active advocacy role.

McKinney claimed that while "we have been trying to limit our focus to gay and bisexual men," the new needs that arose could not be ignored. "It may be that we will get the programs started and then others will take them over," he said, "But I don't think other educational institutions and service agencies will make changes in time to address the need." In that sense, GMHC hopes to become trainers of trainers and pass its wealth of experience and resources on to others.

Because of the urgency of the AIDS situation, GMHC has had to design programs and implement them immediately. For example, the 800 Men Study was conducted in 1985 to test a variety of education interventions designed to teach gay and bisexual men about safer sex. Even though the final results of that study were not released until early 1987, GMHC's AIDS Prevention Program, based on that study, was implemented in January 1986. Funded by the New York State AIDS Institute, the study was the largest and most comprehensive of its kind to date, and the results verified the validity of the program. But GMHC decided to risk implementing the program a year before its results were known, thereby possibly saving hundreds of lives.

Another difference between GMHC and other AIDS organizations is the agency's funding base. Even today more than half its operating budget comes from private sources. According to GMHC's Raymond Jacobs, "We are expected to care for 75%

of the people with AIDS in New York City, yet the City only gives us 13% of our operating budget." It is community support that has made GMHC a viable and growing organization.

One of the biggest controversies surrounding GMHC today is its name. Jacobs explained:

We were formed by a group of gay men who were responding to an unknown killer disease in their community. We have chosen to keep the words "Gay Men's Health Crisis" as our title because those are the roots from whence we've come. Even though 30% of our clients and more are non-gay, we still think it is important to keep our title. Part of our mission is to educate the public that being gay doesn't mean we are different. By being "Gay Men's Health Crisis" and being who we are and succeeding at what we are succeeding at, we are reducing homophobia.

Yet the word "gay" in the organization's title has denied the agency direct access to the high schools and junior high schools, for instance. Even though there has been some informal contact with schools and youth agencies, and even though those groups have come to GMHC for resources and guidance, it is unlikely that GMHC will be able to officially educate in these settings for some time to come.

The African-American and Latino communities, which have been extremely hard hit by AIDS in New York City (as in other large cities), have often been critical of GMHC. The criticism comes from two opposing directions. GMHC is criticized, on the one hand, for not trying hard enough to reach these communities, and on the other hand, for presuming to try to reach these communities despite being a largely white, gay, middle-class, male agency. Both sets of critics agree that GMHC has not done enough to share its expertise and resources with organizations serving IV drug users, Blacks, Latinos, and women.

GMHC continues to debate how to use its limited resources to meet unlimited needs. That the agency has the longest experience and most direct access to the gay and bisexual community in New York City is beyond question. Perhaps Dr. McKinney best summed up the dilemma when he said:

The fact that we're gay has had a great deal to do with the success we've achieved. The kind of commitment to a cause is far greater because we were discriminated against as gay people. Despite the fact that there were those who denied their support to us, perhaps because we were gay, I don't think that we are capable of that same lack of sensitivity toward humanity.

Richard Dunne, executive director of GMHC, feels that what makes GMHC different from other AIDS organizations is that GMHC has a national focus. "The access to and ability to use the [national] media is an important part of the educational function of the organization." Because of its age and reputation, GMHC has a national visibility that other organizations do not have.

Some of the issues on which there is now national focus (e.g., HIV antibody testing and contact tracing) are issues on which GMHC's position will influence other agencies across the nation. Dunne discusses the fine dividing lines between advocacy, lobbying, and education as GMHC takes a position on an issue:

I'd say it's education because we engage in a dialogue. We don't have fixed positions on these things. We try to learn from other people and we hope they learn from our experience. Advocacy assumes you've already made up your mind on these issues. Lobbying has not only a particular view, but is specific to the point of view of funding or a specific law or the wording of the law.

Dunne points out that AIDS education is changing, however. He agrees that GMHC's main focus has been gay and bisexual men and that this focus will necessarily widen as time goes on. "What has changed is that we share or compete with many, many other organizations that are getting involved." GMHC's mission will remain the same, he said, but another role will be added to that of educator: to help ensure that nationally distributed education materials meet professional standards.

The infusion of money into AIDS education which is beginning to happen, as it happened with medical research a few years ago, will draw people into AIDS education who are not in it now or who have not been in it for very long. Generally we applaud that. However, there are some what I call opportunistic entrepreneurs. Government money is now going out on contract to people whose motivation is a lot different than the people who have been motivated to get involved up to this point.

Dunne viewed this as a potential trouble spot that GMHC would like to watch carefully.

GMHC's educational motto is "Fighting the Fear with the Facts." Its mission is to stop the spread of AIDS. In the words of Dr. McKinney, "If we can get to our target population before the virus does, we can save lives. We can't afford to make compromises."

What Gay and Bisexual Men Know About AIDS

Gay and bisexual men constitute the largest proportion of people with AIDS. As of late 1988, almost 70% of adult AIDS cases in the United States were among men who had sex with other men. No group has been more devastated by the epidemic, and no group has amassed more experience in educating itself about AIDS and acting to prevent its spread. As a result, all health educators can learn from the gay community's effort to control AIDS.

Beginning in the early years of the epidemic, when AIDS was designated "gay-related immune deficiency," gay men began to mobilize their community against the syndrome and the stigma attached to it. By early 1982, GMHC was founded in New York City. In the same year in San Francisco, the Kaposi's Sarcoma Research and Education Foundation, later renamed the AIDS Foundation, was established; soon thereafter, groups were formed in Los Angeles, Atlanta, Houston, Dallas, and other cities.

Gay periodicals such as the *New York Native*, the *Gay Community News* (Boston), and *The Advocate* (Los Angeles) played an important role in AIDS education, as did the newly formed AIDS organizations. At first, there was little support for AIDS education from outside the gay community, but as Jeff Natter of GMHC observed, "While governmental inadequacy may have meant an initial shortage of funding, ultimately it provided the gay community with an impetus to address its own needs and develop programs specifically designed to speak to a gay audience."

As a result, by the end of 1988, most gay men in large urban areas were very knowledgeable about AIDS. A variety of surveys and research studies suggest the following generalizations:

- High proportions (80 to 95%) of gay men know how AIDS is transmitted, what constitutes high-risk behavior, what the common symptoms are, and what the HIV antibody test means. However, few researchers have looked at differences in knowledge among subgroups of gay men (e.g., Blacks, high school dropouts, adolescents).

- Significant proportions (40 to 60%) of gay men have made some changes in their attitudes toward high-risk sexual activities and in their sexual practices. One indicator of changed behavior is dramatically lower rates of other sexually transmitted diseases (STDs) among gay men.

- Although more than half the men queried in several studies report a reduction in unsafe sexual practices, a significant number continue to engage in unsafe behaviors at least occasionally. For example, many men have reduced their number of sexual partners and use condoms more frequently but still have episodes of unprotected anal intercourse.

What these data suggest for AIDS educators is, on the one hand, a success story of unprecedented dimensions. In only a few years, the vast majority of gay men in urban areas have become knowledgeable about AIDS, and many have made changes in their sexual behavior. Transmission of HIV infection in large urban gay communities has all but stopped. On the other hand, the high prevalence of HIV infection among gay men makes further improvements crucial if the spread of the epidemic is to be stopped. Moreover, limited research on homosexual or bisexual men who do not identify themselves as gay or who do not live in large urban areas makes it difficult to ascertain whether these groups have also been reached by previous education campaigns.

Messages for Gay and Bisexual Men

Steven Morin, a psychologist who works with the San Francisco AIDS Foundation, has suggested five central messages that AIDS educators need to communicate to gay and bisexual men:

- AIDS is a dreadful disease and I am at risk for it or may threaten others with it.

- AIDS is avoidable. Certain actions will reduce the threat of my getting AIDS or giving it to someone else.

- I can manage new low-risk behaviors that will reduce the threat of my getting or transmitting AIDS and I can still lead a satisfactory life.

- I am willing and able to talk to potential sex partners about low-risk behaviors that will lessen the threat of my getting or transmitting AIDS.

- My peers and community will support these new behaviors.

These messages constitute one dimension of a curriculum for AIDS education for gay and bisexual men (and for other risk groups as well). To translate these statements into action requires addressing learners' knowledge, attitudes, and behaviors. It is noteworthy that these messages are equally relevant for those already infected with HIV and those who are uninfected.

A second dimension of AIDS education must address the social and political context in which gay men live. As described in Chapter 1, homophobia (the irrational fear and hatred of lesbians and gay men) has decisively influenced how our society has responded to the AIDS epidemic. Gay organizations involved in AIDS education have insisted that prevention campaigns aimed at gay men must affirm their right to define for themselves a sexuality and a lifestyle that acknowledges and accepts their sexual orientation. As Cindy Patton, former editor of the *Gay Community News,* noted: "Sex is often perceived as the cement in the gay male community: gay men fear that if sexual ties are reduced or deemphasized the community as whole will disintegrate. Without community institutions and support for sexual practice and political action, some men fear that the identity they struggled to create will be destroyed."

Thus, effective AIDS education for gay men must at the same time encourage significant changes in sexual attitudes and behaviors and reject moralistic and negative views of homosexuality. This dilemma is the central paradox facing AIDS educators in the gay community.

Methods of Education for Gay and Bisexual Men

Teaching gay men about safer sex is probably the most common education effort AIDS organizations have undertaken. "We conduct safe-sex parties in people's homes," reported Leslie Kooyman, executive director of the Metroline AIDS Project in Charlotte, NC. "The parties are small, eight to ten men, informal and very upbeat. It is an excellent tool for gay men to discuss AIDS in a nonthreatening environment. They also provide a great deal of prevention information."

The STOP AIDS Project in San Francisco uses a similar approach. Volunteers are trained to facilitate small group discussions, primarily among gay men. These sessions provide participants an opportunity to learn about AIDS, share their feelings about safe and unsafe sex, and examine possible lifestyle changes. Bert Bloom, outreach coordinator for STOP AIDS, explained that the groups are "really about peer counseling, people in the group talking to each other, getting feedback and learning from each other's experiences."

GMHC in New York City has led safer-sex workshops for much larger groups—150 to 300 people. Through the use of a carefully structured format, participants are taken through the steps of mourning the losses imposed by the AIDS epidemic, affirming the erotic potential of safer sex and condoms, discovering specific ways of having satisfying safer sex, and negotiating sex practices with a partner. See Figure 20 for a summary of GMHC's workshop. GMHC stresses the importance of taking a positive celebratory approach toward safer sex; its first posters announced "Healthy Sex Is Great Sex," and a current brochure (see Figure 21) states: "Safer sex is great sex. It can be fun, exciting—hot, horny—and completely satisfying. It is absolutely possible to continue having great sex! Have all the sex you want—just be sure to always make it safer."

GMHC also distributes brochures, comic books, and a safer-sex video in the style of a pornographic film. The film is shown in gay bathhouses because, Raymond Jacobs, coordinator of AIDS prevention at GMHC explained, "Men who have sex with other men but who do not call themselves gay or men who are in the closet tend to frequent bathhouses," making such places an excellent locale for communicating with these hard-to-reach groups.

Organizations conducting safer-sex education programs have discovered that explicit sexual language is needed to communicate risk behaviors clearly. Says Michael Shernoff of GMHC, "For safer-sex education to go on, you have to have it happen in a context that's recognizable to the people who are involved. People are more likely to talk about 'dicks' and 'cum' as opposed to 'penis' and 'semen.' I don't know anyone who thinks about sex as 'anal intercourse' except the doctor—and he's not the one getting fucked." The use of familiar explicit language also provides learners with a vocabulary they can comfortably use in sexual negotiations in bars and in their bedroom.

Most gay organizations have produced safer-sex pamphlets, some in a format that could be carried in a wallet or pocket. An example is illustrated in Figure 21. Occasionally, explicit language has created

Figure 20. OUTLINE OF GMHC SAFER-SEX WORKSHOP*

GOALS

The goals of the workshop are:

1. To provide participants with a safe, structured, supportive and non-threatening group experience where they can explore and discuss emotionally laden material about AIDS and sex.
2. To help gay and bisexual men identify negative affective responses induced by the AIDS crisis in relation to their sexuality and sex lives.
3. To help participants work through these negative feelings to minimize any impairment in their psychosocial/psychosexual functioning.
4. To help participants see their reactions as appropriate responses requiring new crisis management skills.
5. To help participants discover and share information on how to be sexually active in low-risk ways.
6. To help participants improve levels of sexual health and functioning.
7. To help participants gain practice in negotiating and contracting around safer sex.

CONCEPTUAL FRAMEWORK

The workshop is structured in four therapeutic parts.

I. Mourning
The participants are given the opportunity to express their feelings about the changes they must make if they are to remain sexually active in a responsible way during the AIDS crisis. They learn that they are not alone in these feelings. They are helped to recognize the need to mourn the loss of old sexual patterns and the loss of being able to act on sexual impulse.

II. Affirming
The participants discover that a wide variety of sexual options is still available to them. This part teaches how to degenitalize sex. The focus is to empower participants with a sense of sexual possibility and adventure, as well as the ability to change old patterns.

A major component of this part of the workshop is giving the participants permission to have various thoughts, feelings and actions: to be angry, sad or relieved; to talk about sex; how they might miss high-risk activities; how to be sexual in the face of the epidemic; and how to be erotically playful with a group of other men.

III. Eroticizing
The participants discuss how to eroticize safer options. The focus is to help men let go of thoughts, feelings and actions that are erotophobic, by providing a successful, sex-positive, conceptual experience in a small, non-threatening group setting.

IV. Negotiating
Through role playing and values clarification exercises, the participants learn how to negotiate safer sex agreements and set limits about sticking to safer sex agreements. This increases feelings of self-confidence, thus preparing them to discuss safer sex in future encounters with potential partners.

---

* Excerpted from Palacios-Jimenez L and Shernoff M: *Eroticizing Safer Sex.* New York, Gay Men's Health Crisis Inc., 1986, pp 2, 4.

Figure 21. GMHC BROCHURE ON SAFER-SEX GUIDELINES FOR GAY AND BISEXUAL MEN

Safer sex is great sex! It can be fun, exciting—hot, horny—and completely satisfying. It is absolutely possible to continue having great sex!

Who is at risk for AIDS?
Guidelines for safer sex should be followed by everyone. Anyone who is sexually active is at risk of exposure to the AIDS virus. The only exception is the couple who has been in an exclusively monogamous sexual relationship since 1978. To date, gay and bisexual men, IV drug users, and their sexual partners have been most affected by the disease.

Because many people already carry the AIDS virus (especially in New York City and other major urban areas), reducing the number of different sexual partners does not guarantee safety from exposure. All it takes is one infectious partner for exposure. But even if one has been exposed it is thought to be important to avoid repeated exposure to the virus.

Risk reduction practices must always be followed in every sexual encounter. ***Have all the sex you want—just be sure, always, to make it safer.***

AIDS is transmitted through the exchange of ***certain*** body fluids—you ***cannot*** get AIDS from casual contact (hugging, kissing, sharing bathrooms and kitchens).

The exchange of *cum* (semen) and *pre-cum* should be avoided:

- **In oral sex**
  —Avoid putting the head of the penis into your mouth.
  —Never allow anyone to ejaculate into your mouth.
  —Use a condom for the greatest freedom in oral sex.
- **In anal sex**
  —***Always*** use a condom, with water based lubricants such as KY®. Some experts encourage the use of spermicidal jelly containing Nonoxynol-9.
  —Withdrawing before ejaculation, even with a condom, is safest, since a condom can break.
  —Under no circumstances should you ejaculate semen into the anus.
- **In vaginal sex**
  —***Always*** use a condom. If you use a lubricant, it should be water based, such as KY®.
  —Withdrawing before ejaculation, even with a condom, is safest, since a condom can break.
- **The exchange of *blood* should be avoided:**
  —***Fisting is dangerous!*** And carries the risk of AIDS transmission through the exchange of blood. If you do it, always use a rubber glove.
  —If you inject drugs, never share needles, cookers, or other drug paraphernalia.
  —If you are bisexual, avoid contact with menstrual flow. Use a condom.
- **What about *saliva*?**
  —The virus has been isolated in saliva, though rarely, and in very low concentration. The exchange of saliva is generally thought not to be a risk for AIDS.
- **What about *urine* and *feces*?**
  —Although the virus could theoretically be present in any body secretion, urine, feces, sweat and tears are not known modes of transmission. Oral contact with fecal matter (rimming) should be avoided to reduce the risk of other sexually transmitted diseases. One should use a condom, finger cot, or rubber glove, if giving rectal massage. Avoid oral contact with fingers after this.

Alcohol and **drugs** may impair your judgment and may compromise your immune system. **Poppers** (inhalants) have been linked to Kaposi's Sarcoma, a cancer associated with AIDS. DON'T USE POPPERS.

Mutual masturbation, hugging, frottage (body rubbing), cuddling, showering together, and massaging do not involve the exchange of body fluids, and therefore are considered safe.

Ultimately, practicing safer sex is a personal choice. These guidelines will help to give you enough information to make responsible choices.

Be creative. Enjoy Safer Sex! For further information, call the GMHC Hotline: 212-807-6655. The Safety Pin. The Symbol of Safer Sex. Show you care about Yourself and Your Partner.

conflict with government funders opposed to "obscene" language or to visual representations of human genitals. AIDS educators in Boston, Los Angeles, Charlotte, NC, and elsewhere reported they had to withdraw publications they produced or change the language in order to be able to use government funds for printing. "There's no doubt government rules on what we can and can't say have made our job harder," said one educator.

Most groups also believe that gay organizations and individuals are best suited to do education in the gay community. Unlike much traditional sex education, in which a powerful group seeks to convince a less powerful group of the morality of its sexual preferences, Jeff Natter of GMHC explained that "because [GMHC safer-sex] guidelines have been devised, edited, and circulated by gay men for gay men, the power dichotomy is largely undercut. Those who hear the guidelines do so knowing that those who present them are coming from similar backgrounds and grappling with similar issues of health and sexuality."

To help ensure that gay men practice safer sex, AIDS organizations have also distributed condoms in bars, bathhouses, and elsewhere. An AIDS educator in Pittsburgh reported that one of the most encouraging signs of the impact of education programs was the "male hustlers who keep returning for condoms."

Safer-sex educators face a variety of obstacles in carrying out their work—obstacles involving their own feelings and attitudes, attitudes of the learners they work with, and larger social and political barriers. These obstacles, and some potential solutions, are summarized in Figure 22.

A major problem is the enormity of trying to change behaviors deeply rooted in the culture and value system of gay men. Repeatedly, educators must face up to the realization that providing information is not enough. A gay AIDS educator working in San Francisco explained this issue in personal terms. "Knowing about safer-sex guidelines doesn't mean you're going to do anything about it. There are some things in the unsafe category that I really like to do, so every time I have sex it's a real conscious effort not to do those things. But what choice do I have? I want to survive."

Some educators report that, paradoxically, this problem increases as the epidemic spreads. In earlier years, AIDS organizations reached primarily the most motivated and concerned individuals, those who were already considering making changes. Bert Bloom of San Francisco STOP AIDS noted, "Now we're getting the hard-core people who for the last five years managed to deny AIDS. Reluctantly, they're beginning to realize their risk." Bloom explained that the longer they work at educating, the harder it becomes to educate. This observation demonstrates that it is not true that AIDS education in the gay community is no longer necessary. In fact, more resources and new efforts will be needed to reach less-motivated sectors of the community.

A second goal of AIDS education in the gay community has been to mobilize and organize people to advocate for more resources for AIDS prevention, research, and treatment and against discrimination toward gay men and lesbians. In Washington, DC, in June 1987, 64 demonstrators (some with AIDS) were arrested in front of the White House in a protest against the Reagan Administration's AIDS policies. Earlier that same day, AIDS activists booed and hissed then Vice-President George Bush after he endorsed President Reagan's call for mandatory HIV testing.

In April 1983, GMHC organized a circus benefit performance in New York City. More than 18,000 people, including New York City Mayor Edward Koch, attended. However, the *New York Times* did not

Figure 22. PROBLEMS FACING AIDS EDUCATORS WORKING WITH GAY OR BISEXUAL MEN, AND SOME POSSIBLE SOLUTIONS

Problem	Possible Solutions
Problems Related to Personal Characteristics, Attitudes, or Feelings of Educators	
Discomfort talking about sex.	Institute staff training. Recruit staff with expertise in sex education.
Negative attitudes toward gay men.	Confront attitudes through peer discussion or support groups. Institute special training to sensitize staff or volunteers.
Perceptions by people of color, women, or gay/bisexual men of negative attitudes by white, male, or heterosexual staff or volunteers.	Recruit people of color, women, and gay men as staff and volunteers. Institute training for staff and volunteers to overcome biases.
Need for support because of grief, loss, and the enormity of the epidemic.	Develop informal peer support and structured groups in the organization. Encourage staff to use mental health services.
Staff perception of personal risk from AIDS.	Confront attitudes through open discussion with peers. Institute training or support groups to deal with these feelings.
Unfamiliarity with language, culture, or values of gay men or subgroups of gay men.	Build linkages with other groups already working with or familiar with gay community. Hire educators familiar with culture. Institute training on gay culture.
Problems Related to Knowledge, Attitudes, or Behavior of Learners	
Denial of risk or belief that AIDS is only a problem for others.	Repeat information on risk. Use people with AIDS who are similar to audience as educators. Demonstrate specifically how people can reduce risk.
Unwillingness to change risky behavior.	Concentrate on individuals or groups who are willing to change. Offer options for change (e.g., if you do not want to give up certain sex practices, learn how to make them safer). Reduce or minimize barriers to change (e.g., condom comfort workshops).

Figure 22. PROBLEMS FACING AIDS EDUCATORS WORKING WITH GAY OR BISEXUAL MEN, AND SOME POSSIBLE SOLUTIONS (cont.)

Problem	Possible Solutions
Problems Related to Knowledge, Attitudes, or Behavior of Learners (cont.)	
Opposition or unwillingness to discuss sexual behavior.	Confront unwillingness head on. Distribute literature for people to review in private. Discuss sex in context of learner's culture and values.
Negative attitudes toward people with AIDS.	Repeat message that AIDS is not spread by nonsexual social contact. Focus blame on virus rather than on individuals. Use people with AIDS as educators.
Learners are illiterate or semiliterate.	Develop materials for people with low reading level. Rely on verbal communication and participatory exercises.
Problems Related to Social and Political Factors	
Discrimination against gay men and lesbians.	Use AIDS as a way to confront these attitudes. Build or join coalitions to oppose discrimination.
Political and religious opposition to sexually explicit education about AIDS.	Accept limitations and work around them. Make explicit statement about how limitations undermine public health campaigns.
Restrictions on how government funds can be used for AIDS education.	Understand the boundaries of what is acceptable and create programs that will not challenge them. Seek other sources of funding for controversial programs. Join or form coalitions to oppose restrictions. Comply with restrictions formally but find ways to do what needs to be done (e.g., state importance of abstinence but still teach safer-sex techniques).

cover the story. Several groups protested: The *New York Native* ran a story under the headline "The Greatest Blackout on Earth," and GMHC organized a picket line at the *New York Times* offices. Eventually the executive editor wrote a letter of apology, and coverage of AIDS in the *New York Times* improved somewhat, though it was nearly four years before it began regular coverage of the impact of the epidemic on the city.

These incidents illustrate how gay organizations have used protests and mass media to educate their own community and the larger society about AIDS. Most observers agree that this education and mobilization has played a vital role in both increasing knowledge about AIDS and winning new resources for AIDS prevention.

Creating a Culture of Prevention

The overall impact of individual efforts at safer-sex education and political organization is greater than the sum of its parts. Together, these activities strengthen and reinforce each other to create a culture that supports and encourages preventive action. How does this happen?

First, political mobilization leads to increased self-esteem for individuals who feel they can be actors rather than passive subjects. This is particularly important for a stigmatized group such as gay men. Mobilization can also lead to stronger community organization, which increases the likelihood of winning additional resources for AIDS prevention in the political arena.

More resources create the possibility for more education and therefore a better-informed population. An educated population, one that has the potential to make choices about behavior, is more likely to reduce risky behaviors. Changes in behavior in one sector of the population create peer support for innovation, leading to further reductions in risky activities.

These hypothesized relationships are shown in Figure 23. Although this schema simplifies a complex reality and does not address powerful obstacles, it does provide a framework for multifactoral intervention. Gay organizations have made a conscious effort to coordinate their educational and advocacy work to make the most of the impact. GMHC, for example, tries to develop messages that support cultural change.

Figure 23. RELATIONSHIPS BETWEEN POLITICAL MOBILIZATION AND EDUCATION

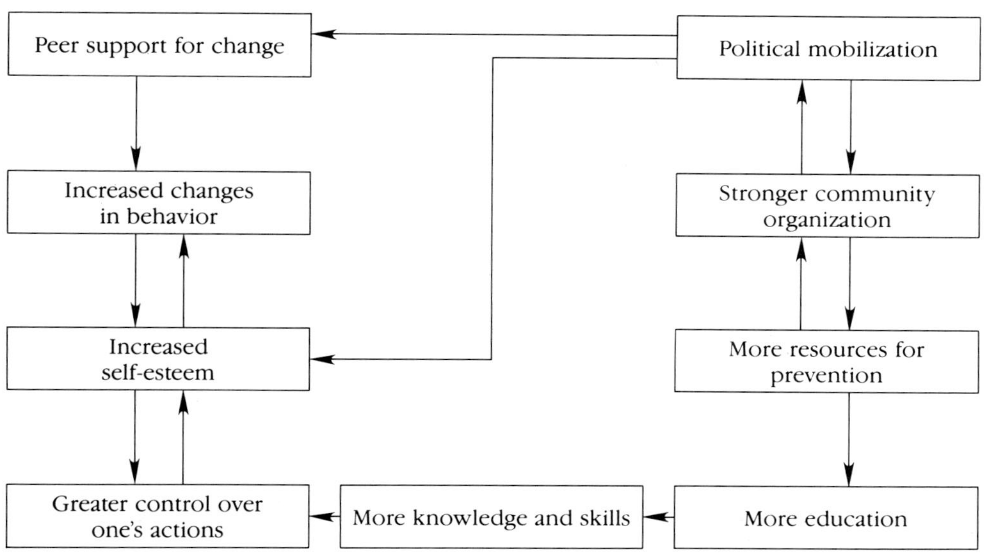

"Rubbers are bringing men together again" is written on condom packages GMHC distributes, emphasizing condoms as a positive tool to reclaim the sexuality threatened by AIDS.

GMHC also sponsored a contest in the gay community to choose a symbol for safer sex. The winner was a safety pin. As Jeff Natter noted, safety pins are inexpensive and readily accessible. Their very name reinforces the notion of safety and provides a degree of wit and playfulness. Now most GMHC literature carries a logo of a safety pin. At the Gay Pride Parade in New York City in 1986, GMHC volunteers carried yard-long silver-color safety pins, thereby (as Natter observed) "elevating the image from symbol to icon in the eyes of hundreds of thousands of parade viewers."

When thousands of gay men wear safety pins, they announce to the world that they are gay and proud of it and that they practice safer sex. The pin offers potential sexual partners the opportunity to either discuss sexual preferences or short-circuit such discussion because of the shared assumption that any sexual behavior will follow safer-sex guidelines.

The opposition of many gay organizations to policies such as closing gay bathhouses and mandatory HIV antibody testing for certain sectors of the population also combines a political and a behavioral focus. Politically, gay activists insist that gay men themselves must define a sexuality that is health promoting; no one can impose that from the outside. Thus, closing bathhouses deprives many gay men of an important outlet for both social and sexual interactions. When the government closes bathhouses, it limits its opportunity to continue to provide credible education; bathhouses offer an ideal education forum for hard-to-reach gay and bisexual men. Similarly, mandatory testing can reinforce the idea that individuals who are not infected need no longer worry about their sexual behavior. It can also drive people in need of education away from the health care system.

In sum, what AIDS organizations in the gay community have accomplished is the establishment of an open dialogue on individual and community responsibility for sexuality, health, and freedom. Individuals need and want information to participate in this dialogue and, in participating, contribute to the momentum for changes in risky behavior, norms, and values. AIDS educators working with other populations will do well to study these accomplishments carefully.

Recommendations

The following recommendations and lessons summarize some of what AIDS educators working in gay communities have learned:

- AIDS educators cannot assume that education is no longer necessary in the gay community. Continual repetition and reinforcement of basic messages is vital. Additional emphasis must be placed on always practicing safer sex, given the high rates of HIV infection among gay men.
- Men who have sex with other men are not a homogeneous community. Educators must identify subgroups of gay and bisexual men and the appropriate channels of communication and messages for each subgroup. See Figure 24 for a list of various sectors of gay men and suggestions on how to reach them.
- Educators working outside the gay community cannot assume that all their learners are heterosexual. Those working with youth, minorities, drug users, prisoners, or any other group must develop education programs that meet the needs of the men in these groups who will have sex with other men.

Figure 24. SUBGROUPS OF GAY AND BISEXUAL MEN AND SUGGESTED LOCATIONS FOR EDUCATION PROGRAMS

Group	Where to Reach
Gay men in mutually monogamous relationship for more than ten years	Not at risk through sexual behavior.
Street youth, hustlers	Runaway centers, youth programs, juvenile detention centers, streets, schools, colleges, sex industry settings.
Young men experimenting with sexual identity	Schools, colleges, street, community.
Married gay or bisexual men	Bathhouses, general media, workplace programs.
"Swingers"	Swinging clubs, swingers' media.
Gay IV drug users	Drug programs, streets, correctional system.
Street cruisers	Street, gay media, bathhouses, bars, sex industry settings.
Gay men who know they are HIV-positive	Health centers, test sites, or community programs for HIV-positive men or people with AIDS.
Gay men with AIDS or AIDS-related complex (ARC)	Hospitals, health centers, or AIDS support organizations.
Gay men of color	Community organizations, Black, Latino, or gay media, churches, workplaces.
Gay prisoners	Prisons, court system.
Prisoners who have sex with other men	Prisons, correctional system.

- All AIDS education programs for gay men must acknowledge the discrimination they encounter in this society and provide learners with tools to combat it.
- Planners of education programs for gay men must include gay men in program development, implementation, and evaluation.
- Safer-sex educators should provide clear and explicit descriptions of sexual behaviors that are safe and risky. It is not enough to say "avoid exchange of bodily fluids." By providing learners with a spectrum of sexual behaviors that are safe, educators leave them with choices to make.
- Safer-sex educators working with gay men must confront their own feelings about homosexuality.

CHAPTER SIX

Intravenous Drug Users

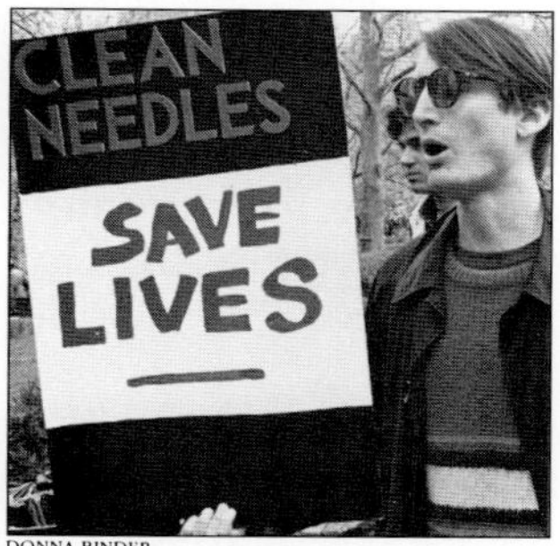

DONNA BINDER

CASE HISTORY

The Community Health Education Project, New Jersey State Health Department

By late 1985, IV drug users and their sexual partners constituted more than half of the reported cases of AIDS in New Jersey, more than three times the proportion for the country as a whole. Two cities in the state, Jersey City and Newark, have the third- and fifth-highest rates of AIDS, respectively, in the United States.

These statistics led state health department officials to focus their AIDS education efforts on IV drug users and their partners. They realized that traditional methods of health education might not be the most effective way of reaching this population.

"The addict population is so difficult to reach," explained Bob Baxter, coordinator of the New Jersey Community Health Education Program for IVDUs. "It's mostly inner city and minority, and they're not going to come to your office for education, they're not going to read your brochures." Baxter believes that creative, community-based interventions that offer more than simple antidrug messages are more likely to be successful in getting the attention and trust of drug users.

Members of the Division of Narcotic and Drug Abuse Control at the New Jersey State Health Department developed a street outreach program because they believed that the most effective way to reach users and their partners would be to get out into the community where the users are—to parks, street corners, and "shooting galleries" (places where addicts can rent needles and inject themselves or be injected).

Baxter described the program as "a very 1960s idea. Those of us who planned this program share the concept of reaching out to IVDUs through their community. This idea was really effective in the 1960s, but when the government cut back on funding, these programs all collapsed. We realized the only way we're going to get to the users is to get back out into their communities and get some street workers like we used to do."

The program planners also believe that ex-addicts are the best candidates for the job of street outreach workers. "The advantage of using ex-addicts is obvious," explained Kristy Lowe, an educator with the state program. "Ex-addicts know the streets, they know where the users are and how to relate to them. They know the language. This is knowledge that you can't get out of a book or some training. They've been there. So they go to places where I, as a professional health educator, can't go."

The outreach workers spend most of their time out in the community talking to people about AIDS and how to avoid HIV infection by adopting safer sexual behaviors and cleaning drug paraphernalia. They also distribute coupons that can be redeemed for 21 days of free detoxification at a state-funded clinic. (Since the Reagan budget cuts of 1981, methadone programs in New Jersey began charging for detoxification services, a policy that led to a 65% decline in the number of people receiving treatment annually between 1980 and 1984.)

Greg Howard, one of the street workers hired by the department to work in Newark, reported a brisk business for coupons. "People are scared," he said. To ensure that detoxification programs educate their clients about AIDS, the state health department requires clinics to document education on the medical record before it will reimburse the program for the coupon.

In addition to the fieldworkers, the state hired experienced health professionals to work in selected drug treatment programs as AIDS coordinators. According to Baxter, "The idea for the coordinators developed because there were so few community organizations getting involved in AIDS in any way. We needed someone to coordinate efforts and to raise the consciousness of the average citizen."

Like the outreach workers, the AIDS coordinators are hired and directly supervised by the drug treatment program in which they work. Technical support is also provided by the state health department. AIDS coordinators are responsible for developing ongoing education regarding AIDS for clients and drug program staff; coordinating services for clients with AIDS or ARC; assuring that support services for people with AIDS are appropriate for clients who are IV drug users; and networking with community agencies to develop coordinated AIDS education programs. Public health nurses, community organizers, and health educators have all been hired to serve as AIDS coordinators.

AIDS coordinators face a variety of problems. Those who do not come from a drug treatment program are often viewed with suspicion by clients and staff. According to Baxter, "Many treatment programs just don't want to deal with AIDS. They don't want to identify with it or be identified as being interested in it." To respond to these attitudes, AIDS coordinators often organize health fairs at which they provide AIDS information.

In a related program, the health department sends out health vans to communities with high rates of drug use. Staff distribute literature, do physical examinations, and encourage people to sign up for treatment programs. By offering general health care, the department hopes to reach and educate people who might not respond to a categorical AIDS program.

How successful are New Jersey's efforts? "It's hard to evaluate a program like this," said Baxter. "You can't go out and see if fieldworkers are really doing what they should because you'll scare off people or you'll get hurt."

Preliminary program data suggest some significant accomplishments. Surveys at intake units of methadone programs show that 70% of those entering treatment report contact with a fieldworker. Of the first 1,000 coupons distributed by outreach workers, 80% have been redeemed. Those who participated in the program showed significant increases in knowledge about AIDS. Given the long latency period for HIV infection, the real effects of New Jersey's program will not be known for years. But as Baxter pointed out, "If every million dollars of prevention efforts saves only seven or eight lives, given current estimates of lifetime costs for caring for a person with AIDS, the program will be cost-effective."

Obstacles to Education Among IV Drug Users

Intravenous drug users constitute the second largest group of people with AIDS in the United States, accounting for nearly 20% of cases. In some areas such as northern New Jersey and (for new cases) New York City, they make up a majority of cases. Preventing the spread of HIV infection through IV drug use is a major goal of AIDS educators. For a variety of reasons, however, this task is particularly difficult.

Negative attitudes toward drug users permeate our society. "In my experience," wrote Pete Hamill, a liberal New York journalist, "junkies don't think of anyone else on earth except themselves and their habits. They will rob their mothers, destroy their families, turn their women into whores, pass their habits on to others to make a few dollars pushing. Why should they suddenly start caring about giving other people AIDS?" A poster displayed in Harlem asks, "When will all the junkies die so the rest of us can go on living?"

This view of addicts as despicable and expendable colors every effort to educate them. Many health care workers do not want to treat addicts; public officials do not want to allocate resources for drug treatment or prevention, and law enforcement agents want to lock them up.

Negative social attitudes toward drug users reflect in part a response to addicts' criminal and antisocial behavior and in part a tendency to blame the victims of social pathology. IV drug users are primarily poor Black and Latino men. By the end of 1988, 80% of people with AIDS related to IV drug use were Black or Latino. Thus, prejudice against drug users intersects with racial prejudices despite the fact that other addictive substances such as cocaine and alcohol are widely used by whites as well. The prevalence of IV drug use in African-American and Latino communities cannot be separated from larger social problems of poor schooling, unemployment, inadequate housing, and poverty. These links to broader inequities make many people feel that addiction is an insoluble problem, reinforcing the tendency to write addicts off. Moreover, addicts can internalize these negative attitudes, further complicating preventive measures. "Developing a sense of social accountability is terribly difficult in a group that does not have a great sense of its social role," noted Dr. Jack Rutledge, deputy commissioner of the New Jersey State Health Department.

Several characteristics of the drug user subculture further hinder education efforts. Because possession and sale of drugs are illegal, and because many drug users must steal, sell drugs, or engage in prostitution or other criminal activities to support their habits, the drug culture is defined as deviant. Drug users often perceive the dominant culture as hostile and view public authorities as adversaries. Hence, any attempt by government or health care providers to convince drug users to change their behavior may be viewed as one more effort to suppress their culture or lifestyle.

To protect themselves against arrest, drug users have developed their own jargon and channels of communication. Because written records could be used as evidence against them, and because some addicts have poor reading and writing skills, most communication is oral. Educators unfamilar with this language or culture will have difficulty reaching drug users. Written materials that do not understand this culture are unlikely to be effective.

Unlike the gay community, which at least in large cities is aboveground and well served by a variety of media, drug users do not have their own media. Surveys in New York City and northern New Jersey show that many addicts do learn about AIDS from newspapers and television, but these messages tend not to address the specific concerns of drug users. Drug users are also susceptible to media inaccuracies and distortions.

Drug-using behavior is deeply rooted in the drug subculture. Samuel Friedman and his colleagues from Narcotic and Drug Research Incorporated (NDRI), a unit of the New York State Division of Substance Abuse Services, noted:

> *The sharing of. . . needles and syringes. . . serves both social bonding and economic functions. Sharing among "running partners" can symbolize their cooperative efforts to obtain drugs. Thus, efforts to reduce sharing works may encounter strong opposition from partners who feel their strongest friendships are under attack or who may need to share works to avoid withdrawal symptoms.*

Although addicts may share drugs and works with a small group of buddies, the general climate is one of mistrust, competition for drugs, and fear of informants and arrest. These attitudes make it difficult to develop a counterculture that emphasizes prevention and mutual responsibility.

Drug users may also find it difficult to accept AIDS as a particularly salient threat. Even before AIDS, deaths from infectious diseases, violence, and drug overdose were common. As Bob Baxter noted, "The life of a drug addict is so fraught with danger that AIDS is just one more hassle, an occupational hazard."

Even for addicts who want to stop using drugs, the choices are limited. In New York City, for example, with a conservative estimate of 200,000 IV drug users, only 35,000 treatment slots are available. At any given time, more than 1,000 drug users are on waiting lists that can delay entry up to several months.

And for those who enter a program, prospects for successful treatment are not optimistic. In most programs, fewer than 30% of those who enroll successfully complete treatment and stay off drugs. Some drug experts have recently called for a dramatic expansion of methadone programs to make treatment available for all addicts who want it, and others have urged wider availability of drug-free programs, Narcotics Anonymous groups, acupuncture clinics, and other treatment methods. Any initiative to expand treatment options, however, must be linked with efforts to improve its effectiveness.

Dr. Robert Newman, president of Beth Israel Medical Center, which operates 23 methadone clinics in New York City, has called the failure to make treatment more available "New York's most outrageous scandal." In its final report in 1988, the Presidential Commission on the HIV Epidemic called for spending $1.5 billion a year for 10 years on new drug treatment programs, providing "treatment on demand" at 2,500 new facilities. Others have called for a relaxation of standards for counseling and supportive services for methadone patients in order to lower the cost of detoxification. Educators need to assess the impact that various policy proposals for expanding access to drug treatment may have on the potential for providing AIDS education in these settings.

Laws on drug use can also hinder successful preventive action. In 11 states, including New York, New Jersey, and Connecticut, each with a high prevalence of AIDS associated with IV drug use, the sale of sterile hypodermic needles and syringes without a doctor's prescription is illegal. This encourages drug users to share and reuse needles. It also promotes the use of shooting galleries. Some surveys of the prevalence of HIV antibodies among drug users in different states suggest that these laws may contribute to the rapid spread of the disease.

The New York City Health Commissioner proposed in 1985, and again in 1987, a pilot project to distribute sterile needles to drug users waiting to enter treatment. Public officials, some Black community leaders, and law enforcement agencies were so opposed that the Mayor declared in 1985 that needle distribution was an idea "whose time has not come and, based on the response, will never come." Yet a 1987 public opinion poll of New York City residents showed that 47% of the respondents approved distribution of free needles and syringes. In October 1988, the city instituted a needle exchange program, but because of political opposition the program was located in a neighborhood far from drug users and few used the service. By the end of 1988, only Tacoma, Washington, had a needle exchange program, this one sponsored by a voluntary organization.

Still another barrier is the reluctance of drug treatment programs to address the issue of AIDS. Judy Spiegel, director of training and professional development for AIDS Project LA in Los Angeles, reported: "Instead of wanting training so that they can adequately provide AIDS-related services and counseling to their clients that need it, drug treatment centers want to dump these people on someone else." Bob Baxter of the New Jersey Health Department explained: "Many drug treatment programs don't want to deal with AIDS; it's a nasty subject. They hope if they ignore it, it'll go away." For programs already saddled with a mission they perceive to be nearly impossible—successfully treating addicts—adding another heavy burden can seem overwhelming. And since many drug counselors are themselves former drug users, anxiety about personal risk can contribute to denial.

Because sharing of contaminated needles presents a particularly efficient route for transmitting HIV infection, most AIDS prevention programs have been aimed at IV drug users. By 1988, however, it was becoming apparent that heavy users of crack or rock, a smokeable form of cocaine, were also at risk of HIV infection.

Preliminary research in New York City and San Francisco showed a significant HIV seroprevalence among regular cocaine or crack users.

Several factors are believed to contribute to HIV transmission in the crack-using population:

- Cocaine, heroin, and other substances are occasionally injected in conjunction with smoking crack.
- The frequency of injection is higher for cocaine than for heroin.
- The rates of prostitution to support drug habits, or the direct exchange of sex for drugs, are high among male and female crack users, often in communities where the "johns" may be former or current IV drug users and are thus at increased risk of HIV infection.
- The hypersexuality associated with cocaine can lead to having multiple sex partners.
- The prevalence of syphilis and gonorrhea is high among crack users, perhaps predisposing to HIV infection.

Because there are few effective treatment options for crack addiction, and because crack addicts seem to be a less-organized community of users than heroin addicts, it is particularly difficult to reach them with AIDS prevention programs.

As a result of these obstacles, many AIDS organizations have given up trying to reach drug users. "We're not hitting IV drug users at all," reported an educator from the Central Iowa AIDS Project. "I think we don't even know how to begin, so we don't start." A group in Connecticut reported that, as a volunteer organization, it did not have the time to do the necessary outreach to drug users. Other groups define a narrow mission for reaching drug users. Nashville Council for AIDS Resources, Education, and Support (Nashville CARES, described in the case history in Chapter 3) trained drug treatment professionals but did not attempt to reach IV drug users themselves. But as the New Jersey case history illustrates, some AIDS organizations have developed innovative and creative ways to overcome the obstacles that make reaching drug users difficult. These approaches will be described after a review of the content of AIDS education for IV drug users.

Content of AIDS Education

The starting point of developing effective education programs for drug users is to find out what they know and do not know. Several surveys of drug users in large cities provide some answers. Educators working in smaller cities may need to do some assessment of their own to determine whether these findings are relevant. (See Chapter 3 for information on how to assess education needs.)

Studies of drug users in different settings in New York City, New Jersey, and California suggest these generalizations:

- The vast majority of IV drug users know that one can get AIDS from sharing needles.
- A smaller but still large majority know that unprotected sexual intercourse can spread AIDS.
- Many continue to believe that AIDS can be spread by sharing a drinking glass or other forms of casual contact.
- More than half of respondents in several studies reported changing their behavior to protect themselves against AIDS. Changes included stopping or reducing the sharing of needles, sterilizing needles, and quitting drug use. Smaller numbers reported changes in sexual behavior, including reducing the number of sex partners and using condoms.

- Nevertheless, significant proportions of drug users continue to engage in high-risk behavior. Many of those who still share needles report that they do so not out of ignorance, but either because no sterile needles are readily available when they need them or because they share with close friends or relatives.
- Surveys of those entering treatment programs show that fear of AIDS seems to motivate some addicts to seek treatment.

These data suggest that education programs (including media coverage, no doubt) have succeeded in giving most IV drug users some accurate information about AIDS. These programs have been less successful in motivating lasting behavioral change. Knowledge may be a necessary condition for taking preventive action, but knowledge alone is certainly not sufficient to reduce the risk.

Figure 25 lists facts, behaviors, and skills that will help protect IV drug users from HIV infection. Educators can use this table to determine the content of education programs aimed at drug users. Figure 26 illustrates how drug users can sterilize their injection paraphernalia.

Strategies for AIDS Prevention

AIDS organizations have used four strategies to reach IV drug users and their sex partners: street outreach workers, education in drug treatment programs, one-to-one counseling, and community organizing. These approaches are not mutually exclusive, and many programs combine two or more strategies.

Street Outreach Workers

The New Jersey State Health Department's street outreach workers illustrate how ex-addicts can be used as AIDS educators. Other programs in New York City, San Francisco, and Baltimore have also used this approach. The Health Education Resource Organization (HERO), the Baltimore AIDS organization, sends ex-addicts to visit shooting galleries, community health centers, outpatient departments, churches, bars, show bars, hotels, motels, and other places where drug users or their partners are likely to be found. "At first," said James Shellington, the supervisor of HERO's program, "people don't want to talk to us, but after we've been in an area for a month or so, they start to trust us. . . . Shooting galleries are the hardest to reach," Shellington reported. "We need to convince the houseman we're not trying to put him out of business. Only then will he let us post our brochures." This trust that develops, based on shared experiences, a familiarity with drug users' language and culture, and repeated encounters, lays the foundation for a relationship in which education can take place.

Other advantages of using ex-addicts as educators are that they provide positive and realistic role models for their clients, they know and can often correctly label and respond to the manipulation or rationalization that drug users offer, and they can have both empathy and impatience toward their clients. Professionals may have difficulty combining these qualities.

What problems have programs hiring ex-addicts encountered? Deciding whom to hire has posed a dilemma. On the one hand, ex-addicts have to be close enough to the drug experience to be able to use it appropriately. "For them to be most effective," explained a staff person in one program, "they have to still have their knowledge of the streets; they can't be too far removed." On the other hand, some distance is needed to ensure that they have indeed solved their own drug problem. "You can't take a guy three weeks out of treatment and expect him to be a good

Figure 25. FACTS, BEHAVIORS, AND SKILLS THAT WILL HELP PROTECT IV DRUG USERS FROM HIV INFECTION

Facts

- The virus that causes AIDS spreads when an infected person's blood, semen, or vaginal fluid gets inside your body. It is not spread in other ways.
- Sharing needles or drug works can cause AIDS.
- Sterilizing needles and works can protect against AIDS.
- Contaminated drugs do not by themselves cause AIDS.
- Use of drugs can lead to many health problems other than AIDS, including hepatitis B, endocarditis, and possibly immune suppression.
- Having unprotected sex with an infected person can cause AIDS.
- Condoms used properly can protect against AIDS.
- If a woman is infected with the virus, she can pass it on to her baby during pregnancy.
- People who are infected with the virus may not look sick.
- Even people who look healthy can give you AIDS if they are infected.

Behaviors To Be Encouraged	Related Skills
Stop shooting drugs.	Finding, entering, and completing treatment program.
Don't share needles or works.	Finding, keeping, and using only one's own works.
If you share needles, always sterilize.	Sterilizing needles, using bleach or other method.
Always follow safer-sex guidelines. Use condoms.	Assessing risk of any sex act. Discussing sex with partner. Using condoms properly.
Get your works before you get your drugs.	Finding and using clean works. Planning drug-seeking strategy.
Women and partners who want to have a child should consider getting tested before getting pregnant.	Assessing usefulness of antibody test. Making decisions about reproduction.

Figure 26. HOW TO CLEAN DRUG WORKS*

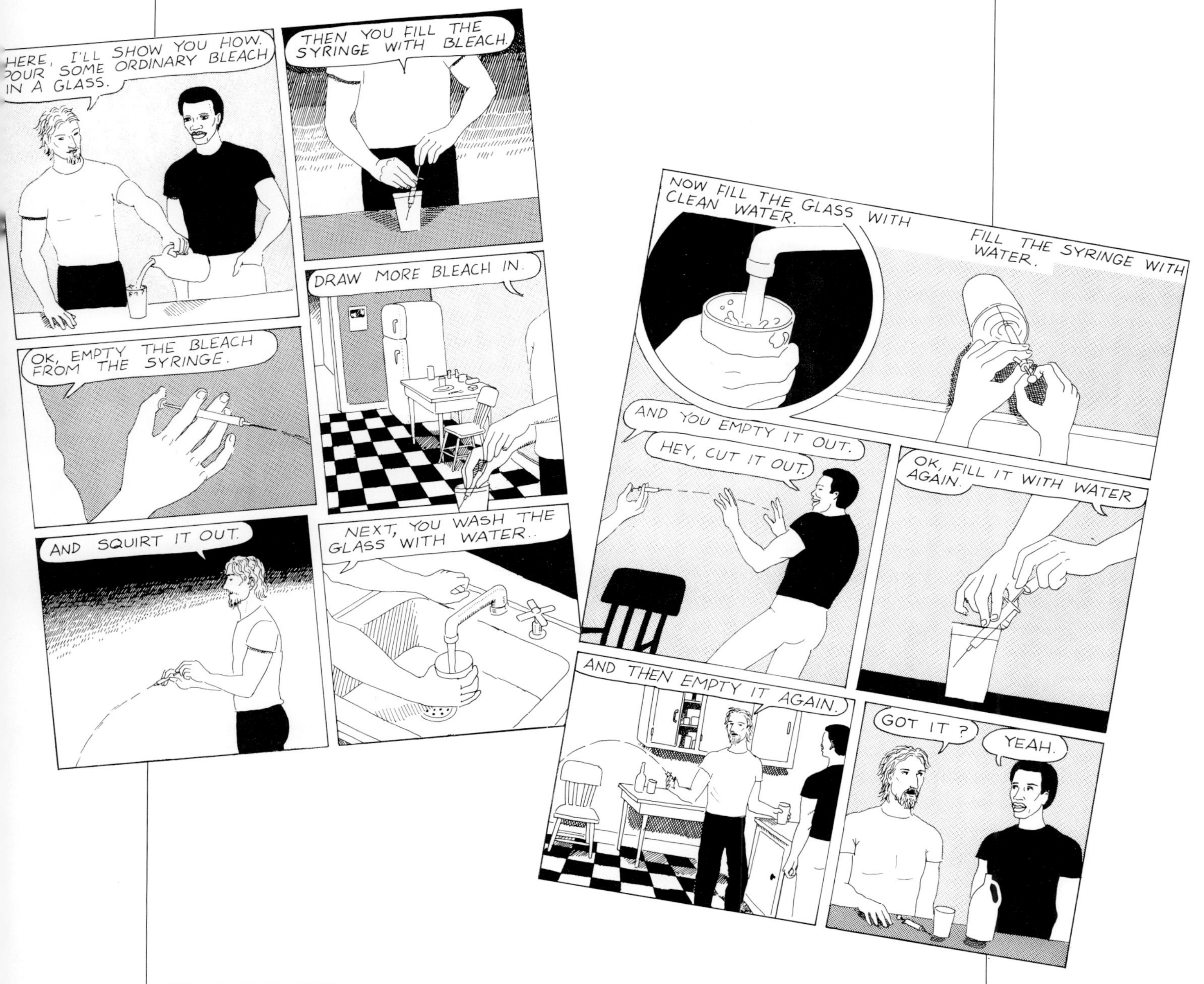
HERE, I'LL SHOW YOU HOW. POUR SOME ORDINARY BLEACH IN A GLASS.
THEN YOU FILL THE SYRINGE WITH BLEACH.
OK, EMPTY THE BLEACH FROM THE SYRINGE.
DRAW MORE BLEACH IN.
AND SQUIRT IT OUT.
NEXT, YOU WASH THE GLASS WITH WATER..
NOW FILL THE GLASS WITH CLEAN WATER.
FILL THE SYRINGE WITH WATER.
AND YOU EMPTY IT OUT.
HEY, CUT IT OUT.
OK, FILL IT WITH WATER AGAIN.
AND THEN EMPTY IT AGAIN.
GOT IT ?
YEAH.

* Excerpted from materials of San Francisco AIDS Foundation. Copyright 1987. Reproduced with permission.

educator," said Bob Baxter. "The odds are he won't even be an ex-addict for long." Most programs insist that ex-addicts must not have used illegal drugs for more than a year. Baltimore's HERO, which hires people still taking methadone, requires 18 months with no illegal drug use and monitors their staff with urine tests.

Supervising ex-addict educators can also be difficult. Baxter noted the problems in checking up on workers in the field. He also observed that he worries about these educators getting into trouble. "They have street smarts, but they also have street egos." One solution is to provide clear guidelines for practice. "I tell my workers that if they don't feel comfortable in a situation, then they don't belong there," Baxter said. "If they're asked to leave, I tell them to just leave because if people don't want you there, they're not going to hear your message anyway." Most programs also tell their staff to notify local police before beginning to work in an area to make sure police officers know what is going on and do not interfere.

Intensive training also helps ensure adequate standards of practice. It gives outreach workers added status both in the community and in the organization. Providing support for outreach workers' own anxiety about their personal risk of AIDS helps ensure that the ex-addicts' personal fears do not interfere with the job.

In summary, hiring ex-addicts to serve as educators and outreach workers provides AIDS organizations with a staff that is likely to communicate effectively with the target population. Careful hiring, close supervision, and adequate training help to ensure that such programs meet their objectives.

Education in Drug Treatment Programs

At some point in their drug-using career, most addicts come into contact with a drug treatment program. Such programs are among the few institutions dedicated solely to drug users and thus provide an ideal opportunity to reach large numbers of IVDUs. Ironically, these programs' low rates of successful treatment emphasize the importance of providing their clients with the information and skills needed to prevent HIV infection. And because many people in treatment programs continue to maintain relationships with other drug users, treatment programs can educate their patients to transmit accurate information to others at risk or who are hard to reach. Finally, the ongoing contact clients have with treatment programs (e.g., several visits a week or a long period of residence) enable continual and intensive education, an option street workers often do not have.

Drug treatment programs have used different methods to reach their clients. Some employ ex-addicts to run education sessions in the facility. Others, like the New Jersey State Health Department program, hire health professionals to provide ongoing education to staff and clients about AIDS. A large drug-free program in New York City brought in consultants to train their existing staff of drug counselors to provide clients with AIDS counseling and risk reduction education.

Many drug treatment programs have resisted adding AIDS education to their mission at first. But some observers believe that with time this reluctance can diminish. Judy Macks, the mental health training coordinator at the AIDS Health Project in San Francisco, reported: "The attitudes in substance abuse facilities have changed in part because more information about AIDS has gotten out, and in part because a year ago these programs might not have seen anyone who was antibody-positive or sick. As soon as you get someone in your program—a real live person who is dealing with AIDS—people want to know how to deal with it."

Educators can use this new-found interest and motivation to help agencies plan how they will respond to the AIDS epidemic. Making the decision to seek education for clients and staff usually raises a host of related questions:

- Will the agency accept substance abusers with AIDS?
- How will it handle enrolled clients who become ill?
- Will it teach its clients how to clean works?
- Will it offer AIDS education to the families and partners of clients?
- Will it distribute condoms?
- What will happen to staff who become ill?

By helping to prepare management, staff, and clients to address these questions, AIDS educators can play a critical role in helping substance abuse facilities define an appropriate role in AIDS prevention.

Individual Counseling

"There's no better way than one-to-one contact to reach drug users who are not in treatment, because the problem with people on the street is that they're not hooked into newspapers, radio, TV, books, and even if they are, they don't trust it in the way they do one-to-one contact," said John Newmeyer, director of education at the Haight-Ashbury Free Clinic in San Francisco.

Counseling allows AIDS educators to assess each learner's specific concern, to get feedback on the interaction, and to develop a personal relationship, all qualities particularly useful in working with drug users. Bryanne Camella, a drug educator with the Boston AIDS Action Committee, reported that when working on the street, she would often approach a group of drug users and offer to provide information on AIDS. Then she would go to a coffee shop with one interested person to talk in depth. "I don't give a talk," she said, "I talk, they interrupt, and then I talk again." This personal style, she felt, was much more likely to lead to real learning than a more formal presentation. Topics covered in counseling sessions include how to find a treatment program, how to clean works, and how to practice safer sex. One-to-one counseling can also be an effective technique for enlisting the sexual partners of drug users in preventive action.

In some cases, counseling is provided in the context of antibody testing. Researchers and clinicians report contradictory findings on the impact of antibody testing on IV drug users. Samuel Friedman of NDRI interpreted the existing evidence to support the view that with adequate counseling, antibody testing can lead to positive changes in drug and sexual behavior for both antibody-positive and antibody-negative drug users. Based on a study of methadone patients treated in clinics in the Bronx, Dr. Peter Selwyn and his colleagues concluded that counseling and education may have been more important in changing behavior than testing itself. They warned that clinicians must anticipate significant psychosocial distress and self-imposed isolation in IV drug users informed of positive antibody status.

Preliminary results from other studies suggest that drug users may respond to the knowledge of their antibody status by increasing risky drug and sexual behavior, at least temporarily. Although more research is needed to assess the impact of testing on drug users, it seems clear that drug users are in great need of extensive pre- and post-test counseling to ensure that testing has a beneficial rather than a detrimental effect. (See "Antibody Testing and Counseling" section in Chapter 4 for a further discussion of these issues.)

Community Organizing and Self-Help

Because drug addiction is a social and political problem as well as a medical one, social and political interventions are appropriate strategies for AIDS prevention. Two examples illustrate this approach.

The San Francisco Mid-City Consortium to Combat AIDS, a coalition of community groups and independent medical clinics, sends volunteers onto the streets to educate drug users and to distribute condoms and 1-oz. bottles of household bleach used to sterilize needles. They also produce cartoon-like instructions on how to use the bleach to clean needles and syringes.

In New York City, the Association for the Prevention and Treatment of Drug Abuse (ADAPT) (an organization of ex-drug users, substance abuse professionals, and some current drug users) seeks both to educate drug users about AIDS and to advocate for the special needs of IV drug users. It also seeks to promote self-organization among drug users.

Self-organization of drug users offers several potential benefits. It provides social support from within the community for users who have adopted less dangerous drug and sexual behaviors. The cumulative impact of individual behavioral changes can lead to cultural changes that support and reinforce prevention, such as a norm of cleaning works before shooting up. This route of change is probably more effective and rapid than one imposed from the outside by professionals. It also permits positive elements of the culture, such as self-reliance and trust between "running mates" (friends who share drugs), to be strengthened and used for prevention. A significant body of literature points to the value of social support in maintaining behavioral changes.

Research also suggests that taking collective action to improve one's living conditions is in itself healthful, contributing to increased self-esteem and perceptions of being in control, and thus leading to decreased drug use. Finally, self-organization can lead to the creation of advocacy groups that can represent the needs of IV drug users in the political arena. The success of gay organizations in winning new resources for prevention and treatment of AIDS points to the power of this strategy.

In some European cities, drug users created their own organizations nearly a decade ago. The Junky League in Amsterdam, for example, set up a free sterile needle exchange, educated addicts about hepatitis B, distributed pamphlets warning about contaminated drugs, and organized to provide improved services for addicts and against police repression.

In the United States, organizations of drug users have emerged more recently. ADAPT, in New York City, conducts community education campaigns, visits shooting galleries and prisons, and enrolls addicts in treatment programs. The organization also trains health professionals and provides a voice for drug users in public debates about AIDS and substance abuse issues. In 1987, ADAPT received a contract for AIDS education among IV drug users from the New York City government, allowing it to hire paid staff for the first time. Yolanda Serrano, president of ADAPT, observed: "Society does not view drug users as being able to organize. They think of [junkies] as uneducable. We feel we refute the stigma that a junkie will always be a junkie. Our members are executives, doctors, lawyers, people you might not think of as drug users. We see ourselves as role models for people using drugs."

Recommendations

AIDS educators working with IV drug users combine the techniques described previously with these recommendations.

- Disseminate widely those facts and behaviors that IV drug users need in order to protect themselves against AIDS (see Figure 25). Using a variety of formats and media to get these messages out will ensure that all sectors of the drug-using population are reached and that reinforcement is provided to those who already know this information.
- Teach the skills needed to achieve the behavioral changes listed in Figure 25. It cannot be assumed that presenting information will by itself lead to change in behavior. Drug users need to learn how to find and enter treatment programs, use condoms, and clean their needles. This requires demonstrating skills, giving learners a chance to practice, and discussing how to overcome the social and psychological obstacles to change.
- Provide ongoing AIDS education for health and social service professionals who come into contact with IV drug users. Health professionals need help overcoming their negative attitudes toward IV drug users. Targeting this group is an effective way to make initial contact with drug users seeking help.
- Educate policymakers and citizens about obstacles to effective prevention, such as lack of treatment facilities and unavailability of sterile needles.
- Target messages to subgroups of drug users as listed in Figure 27. Sexual partners of IV drug users are a particularly important group that can be reached through methods described in this chapter and in the chapters on youth, women, prisoners, and Blacks and Latinos. Former users need information on safer sex, and current users must learn how to clean their works. Young people just beginning to experiment need urgent and intensive help to get off drugs before they become addicted. The health education and social marketing literature suggests that segmenting a population increases the likelihood of effective communication.
- Develop interventions that reinforce positive elements of drug subculture (e.g., trust between running mates) and seek adaptive changes in health. Ex-drug users and self-help organizations are probably best equipped to promote such changes.
- Ensure that every drug treatment program has an active AIDS education component for staff, clients, and their families. Drug abuse staff especially need training in sex education and in coping with their personal risk of AIDS.
- Encourage and support efforts at self-organization among drug users. Health professionals can contribute valuable expertise and access to resources.
- Include safer-sex education in all programs for drug users. Any drug user who is sexually active is at risk of transmitting or acquiring HIV infection.
- Advocate for policies that prevent the spread of HIV infection via drug use.

Figure 27. SUBGROUPS OF DRUG USERS AND WHERE TO REACH THEM

Subgroups	Where To Reach Them
Sexual partners of current drug users.	Health centers, hospital outpatient departments, drug treatment programs, public assistance centers, streets, churches, community agencies, welfare hotels, mass media.
Sexual partners of former IV drug users.	Health care centers, workplaces, all community settings, mass media.
Youth experimenting with snorting or smoking opiates but not yet injecting, or users of crack.	Youth programs, community centers, juvenile detention centers, schools, runaway centers, streets, parks, mass media.
Former users of IV drugs.	Workplace, all community settings, Narcotics Anonymous and other self-help groups.
IV drug users currently in treatment programs— ■ methadone; ■ drug-free; ■ not using illegal drugs; ■ still using IV drugs.	Drug treatment programs, detoxification facilities.
IV drug users currently incarcerated.	Prisons, courts.
Occasional users of IV drugs.	General community settings, streets, schools.
Users who regularly visit shooting galleries.	Shooting galleries, streets.
Users who own and use their own works.	Community settings, places where drugs are sold and used.
Users who want to enter treatment programs.	Intake for treatment centers, streets, community settings, health centers.
Prostitutes (male and female) who use drugs.	Streets, bars, motels, detention centers, sex industry, massage parlors, escort services.
Gay drug users.	Special programs for gay IV drug users; gay media; bathhouses and gay community settings.

CHAPTER SEVEN

African-Americans and Latinos

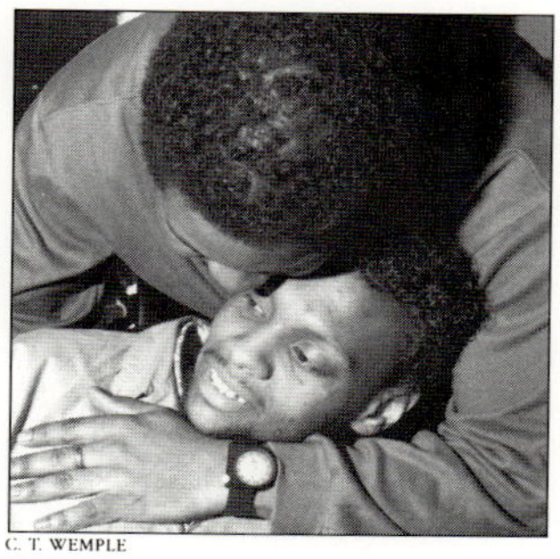

C. T. WEMPLE

CASE HISTORY

Minority AIDS Project, Los Angeles

(an interview with Rev. Carl Bean, Executive Director)

I needed to find out about AIDS because people kept asking me about it. So I went to all of the AIDS organizations in Los Angeles to see what they could tell me. I decided to go through the Shanti Project's training. [The Shanti Project is a California-based organization that provides services to people with AIDS.] During the training, I noticed there were very few people of color, so I asked why. Some told me they had tried to network in "those" communities, but people weren't responsive; others said they didn't know how to network in "those" communities. It seemed that racism was beginning to rear its ugly head.

The more I found out about AIDS and how so many of those affected by it were minorities, the more I began to realize that I had to go back to my community to let them know about this horrible disease. I knew I couldn't be comfortable going out and working with a white organization that wasn't serving the needs of my community. I needed to let my community know that AIDS was a crisis among minorities because they don't know and it's going to get worse because they don't know.

At first, the other groups were supportive. They told me to write a proposal and they would help me start up. That was a total farce. When I went back with my proposal, it was as if I had never been told to create it. They said, "We don't have any money to give you. What do you want to do over 'there'? What do we need to do to get them to come over here?" I kept saying, "Why should we have to go somewhere else to get health care? Why can't we get the same service where we live?"

When I started raising the issue of racism and the lack of concern about AIDS in minority communities, that's when the fireworks began. They wanted to shut me up and thought they could do it by involving me in some token way. But that wasn't enough for me.

I was asked to form a minority AIDS task force for one of the largest AIDS organizations. Now mind you, I had already set up a Minority AIDS Project and I'm the executive director, and I'm supposed to leave that and sit on a task force under their hierarchy to deal with my own community? This made no sense at all!

So they got other Blacks and Latinos to come to this first meeting of this task force. The meeting was stormy. The Blacks and Latinos said, "Well, Reverend Bean has a Minority AIDS Project, and we're already trying to assist him. So if you want to know what you can do to help our communities, help Reverend Bean in what he's doing." We told them that we don't need to go to West Hollywood to sit around and discuss Black and Latino culture. We told them to put the money in the hands of those who are Black and Latino, that they know what to do, so just let them do it. We told them not to do what they usually do—get the money, rush into our communities, turn on a tape recorder, and then think they know enough to solve our problems.

They tried to get around it. Their response was that they realize racism is a problem in America and that parity is a problem, and so on and so on. They actually took out pieces of paper and started listing, "Number 1, racism, number 2, parity," and so on and so forth. They wanted to take 18 weeks to deal with this and 20 more weeks to deal with that. But we kept saying our people are dying now and no one seems to care about getting the message out to them.

By the second meeting, I think that even they knew this was not going to work out. I was supposed to chair the meeting with a woman from the Latino community. This meeting was worse than the last. First, we said we'd hold the meeting in our neighborhood. We held the meeting in a community center in a Black neighborhood. We arranged to have an educational forum on AIDS for IV drug users before the meeting because we wanted to use the gathering to get some information out.

The IV drug users were so attentive. They really wanted to know. They already knew that sharing needles could kill them and they knew the word AIDS, but they really didn't know the how and why. They had so many questions! They knew that we weren't judging them. We only wanted them to have the facts so they could live long enough to change.

After the forum, which was wonderful, the representatives from the white organization came in. They all sat together on one side. One side of the room was white and the other Black and Latino. We asked them, "Don't you see how racist it is for you to think that we should sit under you? That you should be over the money and that you should decide if we can educate our own?"

They said, "Oh no, we're not racist, we don't feel that way." They didn't see the racism inherent in how they wanted to set up this task force to do AIDS education in the minority community. Then they said, "That's why we need to talk more."

We said, "We're not talking any more. We're going to the powers that be to ask for the money to do this work." Their reaction was negative, they didn't like it at all. I told them they were looking at it wrong. We were not going for the piece of the pie that they already have; we're going for the piece of the pie that hasn't been baked. With all the money that those groups have been given, no Black, Latino, or Asian organization concerned about AIDS has ever been included, so we weren't even in the pie! We deserve the same health care and education that the white community is already getting. So we have to have our own money. This other organization thought they were being threatened and then they got the idea to create a minority component to get that money, too.

But we knew this would never work—some satellite clinic in the Black community isn't going to work when it's white directed and controlled. It's whites once again deciding what to do with Black dollars. We've had enough of that.

Even now, it's still felt in many quarters that the large white organizations should still be directing all the AIDS education in this town. And in most cities across the country, they still do.

But now relations with the other AIDS organizations in Los Angeles are friendly enough because they now know we're not going to go away. They thought we would just disappear because we didn't have any money. But it didn't happen like that.

Now we're all working together. We have to. But I can't close my eyes to what America is and how it works. We live in a racist society, and that's true whether we want to look at it or not. With AIDS we're dealing with life and death, so we don't have time to deal with racism workshops and such, because my people are dying.

We may work together, go to school together, but at the end of the day we take buses and freeways in different directions. Because in America, we still live separately. Therefore, when they start carving up money, they carve up Black dollars, white dollars, women's dollars, and Latino dollars.

Let's not act like because the subject is AIDS, that this is not happening. I'm here to tell you I ain't shutting up until the dollars that are supposed to be in my community are there.

So finally, after two years, we've won our first state contract for education in the Black community. Also, we now have a small county contract, and we just applied for a new contract created for underserved minority communities.

Now there is finally money for the things we fought so hard for during the past two years. We strongly believe that money for AIDS education should go to community-based organizations and not to some outside organization that wants to put a Black person in an office and call that their Black outreach office and think that they're doing education. But our kind of education is finally happening.

Obstacles to AIDS Education in African-American and Latino Communities

This chapter focuses primarily on African-American and Latino populations because they are currently most severely affected by AIDS and the recipients of most of the AIDS education programs targeted at people of color. As AIDS educators now doing prevention work with Asian, Native American, and other racial and national groups gain more experience, guidelines for working with these groups need to be developed.

Unlike gay and bisexual men, some of whom are at higher risk of AIDS because of their sexual behavior, or intravenous drug users, some of whose injection practices elevate their risk, African-American and Latino people have no special characteristic as a group that makes them more vulnerable to HIV. Rather, it is specific patterns of drug and sexual behavior that put some Blacks and Latinos at risk. A review of prevalence data leaves no doubt that African-Americans and Latinos are in fact at greater risk of developing AIDS. A few statistics illustrate this point:

- Although Blacks and Latinos accounted for only 20% of the US population by the end of 1988, they constituted 42% of the cases of AIDS;
- Blacks and Latinos volunteering for the US Army are three to ten times more likely to be infected with HIV than white volunteers;
- Black and Latino gay men who do not use IV drugs are 1.6 times more likely to get AIDS than similar white men;
- Black women are 12 times more likely and Latina women 9 times more likely to get AIDS than white women.

Effective prevention programs in African-American and Latino communities must address both the existence of homosexual behavior and drug addiction and the reality of racism and poverty, both of which contribute to the high prevalence of AIDS.

Educators working with Black and Latino people throughout the United States report that denial that AIDS is a problem that constitutes a major obstacle. Part of the cause is lack of information. "I don't see any Black stars getting AIDS, so don't tell me AIDS is a Black problem," a high school student told an AIDS educator in New York City. "Black men in San Francisco still seem to think of AIDS as a white problem," reported an AIDS educator in that city. "They think they'll be okay if they just don't fuck around with white boys." Media coverage of AIDS has contributed to the idea that only white gay men get AIDS.

Another reason for denial is a reluctance to accept yet another overwhelming social problem. "I think Blacks are afraid to speak out for fear of being identified with the problem," said Dr. Wayne Greaves, chief of infectious diseases at Howard University Hospital in Washington, DC. "As if to talk about it means you condone what's happening. Or as if you were betraying yourself to admit there's a problem in the Black community."

Some African-Americans and Latinos believe that AIDS cannot compare to more pressing problems such as poverty, unemployment, racism, infant mortality, lack of housing, and poor schooling and that to emphasize AIDS is to slight these issues or to divert public attention from them.

As in other communities, homophobia and dislike for addicts also make AIDS a difficult issue to address. "I think whites are more open about homosexuality," said Dr. Greaves. "Most of my patients and their families would much rather say they got AIDS from IV drugs, rather than from homosexual acts." And Suki Ports of the Minority AIDS Task Force in New York City observed, "There is not a lot of sympathy for drug users from people who have been victimized by drug-related crime." These attitudes are occasionally reinforced by religious beliefs that see disease as a punishment for immoral behavior.

Mistrust of public authorities compounds the difficulty of communications. Linda Williams, a health educator in Detroit, noted that Black people often view the health department as having police powers, as one more agency seeking to impose its agenda on a community. "How can we trust authorities who have not even taken the trouble to teach us how to read?" asked Ruth Rodriguez of the Hispanic AIDS Forum in New York City. The trust issue works two ways. "If you [the educator] are afraid of the group you're talking to, they can pick up on it and smell a research paper coming. They are not going to respond to you," warned Sunny Rumsey of the New York City Health Department's AIDS Education Unit.

Public health officials cannot, therefore, assume that the "facts" they present about AIDS will be accepted. For example, early media coverage and scientific commentary on a hypothesized African origin of AIDS reinforced mistrust, making many African-Americans feel they were being blamed for yet another social problem. Others continue to believe that the AIDS epidemic is a result of government-sponsored biological warfare experiments.

The overall impact of these and other obstacles is that Blacks and Latinos have received less AIDS education than whites and are less likely to be well informed about the disease. Yet they are also more concerned about AIDS than whites. National and local public opinion polls and surveys have shown the following:

- A 1985 national poll by the *New York Times* and CBS found that 65% of Blacks, compared to 49% of the total population, felt that they knew little or nothing about AIDS.
- A 1987 poll by the Illinois Department of Public Health found that compared to whites, Latinos were more likely to have a personal fear of AIDS; Latinos also tended to have more erroneous beliefs about transmission than Blacks or whites.
- In a study of New York City drug users in 1986, whites were significantly more likely than Blacks and Latinos to have heard of techniques for cleaning works that are believed to kill HIV (i.e., bleach, hydrogen peroxide, alcohol, and boiling).
- In a study of San Francisco high school students in 1985, researchers found that although almost all young people knew about sexual and drug transmission of AIDS, considerably more whites than Blacks or Latinos knew that condoms lower the risk of sexual transmission. Minority youth were twice as likely as whites to believe that AIDS can be spread by touching, kissing, or being near a person with AIDS.
- A study of Black gay men in Detroit in 1985 found that many had difficulty finding information on AIDS. Fewer than 10% identified the primarily white gay AIDS organization as a source of information.
- A 1987 Gallup poll showed that 36% of Blacks compared to 18% of whites were "very concerned" that they will contract AIDS.

Principles for Effective AIDS Education

The foregoing data suggest that a concerted effort is needed to ensure that African-Americans and Latinos have access to the information and skills they need to protect themselves against AIDS. In this section, some principles for effective AIDS education in Black and Latino communities are suggested. They are based on interviews, reviews of case histories, and discussions with educators working in these communities.

Do not assume that all racial or national groups are the same or that any particular community is homogenous.

In their eagerness to reach Blacks and Latinos, public health workers sometimes assume that all are the same. This assumption can be manifested in different ways. Educators can look for *the* way to reach Black or Latino people. "The only way to reach Blacks is through Black churches," some say, or, "You have to get the Catholic Church and Latino celebrities to reach Latinos." Both churches and celebrities are valuable allies, but what of those who don't go to church? What about people living in shelters for the homeless or prisons? What about Black college students? "There is no one way to reach the Black community," insisted Amanda Hamilton-Houston, chair of San Francisco's Black Coalition on AIDS.

Educators also cannot assume that one educational format can reach all racial or national groups. "If you're working with minorities," said one AIDS educator at a conference, "make sure you use little words and don't write anything above a high school reading level." Another educator, who worked in Detroit's Black community, responded angrily, "That's racist. I work with Black health professionals and with college-educated people. We need to find out the specific needs of any group we work with, Black or white. You can't assume all Blacks are uneducated."

Still another dangerous assumption is that if persons of color—no matter what their experience or background—are hired to do education, they will develop appropriate interventions. A white AIDS organization in a large city hired a Black man to coordinate its minority education program. When this individual, who had no background in AIDS or in health, had difficulty implementing a program, management interpreted this experience as confirming how hard it is to reach people of color. As Reverend Bean explained in the case history, reaching a Black or Latino community requires giving genuine control to that community.

By using the needs assessment techniques described in Chapter 3, AIDS educators of all races and nationalities can ensure that they understand both the beliefs and the education needs of their learners.

Effective education must be targeted to the specific group to be reached.

"If you give a Black man and woman an AIDS brochure with two white men on the cover, they'll say, 'This isn't for me,' " said Craig Harris, a health educator with the Spectrum AIDS Education Project, which works in Washington, DC's Black community.

Too often, AIDS educators have used films, brochures, and other materials that were produced for white audiences in Black or Latino communities. And changing the color of the faces on the brochure or translating the words into Spanish is not enough. Literal translations can feed the sense of denial about AIDS that already exists. After reading a pamphlet issued by the health department, a Latino educator in San Francisco commented, "This obviously wasn't developed by Latinos for Latinos."

Effective materials should include language and cultural concepts familiar to the intended audiences. "We don't just translate from English to another language anymore," said Bob Schoonover of AIDS Project Los Angeles. "We're now going through the same process in the Latino communities that we do for our other brochures, talking to people first. We now write separate pamphlets in English and Spanish."

Another example is AIDS educators working with Haitians in the United States. These educators must understand and address cultural taboos against homosexuality, the complex interactions between Catholicism and folk medico-religious beliefs, and the stigmatization Haitians have encountered around AIDS. For many Haitians, the US health care system is itself an alien and threatening institution. Without such understanding, educators will be unable to anchor their messages in their learners' world view.

Some Latino and Asian cultures have two distinct sets of rules for discussing sensitive topics: in public, such issues as sexuality or drug use should not be brought up, but in private, in the family or with peers, much wider latitude is accepted. AIDS educators need to understand these differing rules and seek to use both public and private arenas to advance an appropriate agenda for discussing AIDS.

Another cultural dichotomy can face educators working in communities where young people and older people or recent and long-term immigrants have differing values and behavior patterns. For example, adolescents from the Dominican Republic living in New York City may have more in common with the African-American youth they see in school and on the street than with their parents who grew up in rural villages in the Dominican Republic. AIDS educators can often play a useful role by helping organizations serving Black or Latino communities to define these differences and discuss their implications for effective education.

One way to increase the likelihood of effective targeting is to include representatives of target populations in the planning process. In Detroit, for example, health educators from the city health department requested a meeting with community residents concerned about AIDS to ask for help in developing a program for African-American residents. After preliminary discussions, 12 individuals formed the Community Health Awareness Group (C-HAG) to assist in designing a community AIDS education program. The group included men and women, Black gay and bisexual males, former IV drug users, and prostitutes as well as several people not perceived to be at risk. Most members had previously participated in community organizations. Because the members of C-HAG knew the subculture, the informal networks, and the language of the target populations and were themselves known and credible to these groups, they played a vital role in the program. The health educators identified problem areas and objectives for risk reduction and prevention. C-HAG, in turn, made suggestions for appropriate methods and strategies for involving community residents in the process.

The first step for AIDS educators in African-American and Latino communities is to convince people that they are at risk.

Denial that AIDS is a problem is a common response in all communities. Until people perceive that they are vulnerable, there is little possibility for prevention education or action.

AIDS educators working in Black and Latino communities have used several strategies to achieve this goal. Blacks Educating Blacks About Sexual Health Issues (BEBASHI) in Philadelphia (described in

Chapter 3) began its work by targeting leaders of the Black community for education. By meeting individually with elected officials, ministers, civil rights leaders, and others, BEBASHI's director, Rashidah Hassan, was able to convince Philadelphia's Black leadership that AIDS was indeed a cause for concern. This strategy both increased the number of articulate spokespersons advocating more resources for AIDS prevention and opened doors for BEBASHI to take its message directly to those leaders' constituents. BEBASHI also sponsored training sessions for Black journalists, an important group providing information to the Black community.

Repetition also helps to break through denial. "What we need is massive constant education for this message to get across," said Yolanda Serrano, president of ADAPT in New York City. "It has to be constant, otherwise it's not going to get through."

Another strategy that groups have used is linking AIDS with other African-American health issues. Several Black educators reported that this technique helped break through the stigmatization evoked by homosexuality and drug use. Linda Williams, a Detroit health educator, explained: "In order to minimize the alienation of more traditional sectors of the community, . . . [C-HAG] strongly opposed being labeled as a homosexual or AIDS advocacy group. Rather, they chose to adopt a much broader focus relative to the overall health concerns of the Black community."

One result of this broader focus is that AIDS does not become a moral question. Rather, said Reverend Susan Hopkins, education minister in Washington, DC's Black Shiloh Baptist Church, "it's a question of health and survival. Disapproving of AIDS is like disapproving of alcoholism. It's here. And the issue is that it's taking people away."

It should be noted that in raising the level of concern about AIDS, educators must also seek to reduce fear and misinformation, also prevalent among Black and Latinos. This is best accomplished by providing accurate information, listening carefully to people's specific concerns, and providing a variety of opportunities for open dialogue.

Educators must understand and acknowledge the specific sexual values of each racial and national group.

Sexuality includes sexual behavior, moral values, gender roles, and sexual language. Culture defines how human sexuality manifests itself, and the subtle and not-so-subtle sexual variations among people of color present AIDS educators with a significant challenge.

Gender roles shape how men and women view the world and themselves in it. In turn, this view determines how people respond to sex education. "As a psychiatrist," said Dr. Rafael Tavares, a founder of the Hispanic AIDS Forum in New York City, "I can tell you that, for Hispanics in general, there is a much more rigidly defined sense of what men and women should be. Sex is not something that is commonly discussed, and there's a general sense that, for women, it is improper to be too knowledgeable about it. The more prepared she is to deal with the act itself, the more suspect her virtue is."

Sunny Rumsey, a New York City health educator, explained further: "When you tell a Caribbean woman to tell her man to use condoms, you're going up against a culture that prides children. If AIDS educators can't understand a cultural response the tendency is to ask, 'What's wrong with these people, they're trying to kill themselves.' "

Attitudes toward homosexuality may also differ among people of color. A focus group of Black, Latino, and Asian leaders from San Francisco, discussing how best to reach their communities, concluded that "homophobia was greater within minority subcultures than in mainstream American culture," a view frequently reported by educators working in Black and Latino communities. Although quantitative evidence to confirm this belief is lacking, observers point to the tendency of some Black families to disown gay children who come out of the closet and the pervasiveness of "machismo" within the Latino culture. One participant in the San Francisco focus group explained that in Asian culture, "to be open about AIDS or homosexuality is to raise questions like 'Why is he doing this and bringing shame to his family?' "

African-American and Latino men who have sex with other men may also interpret that experience differently than white men do. "Many minority men who are gay do not identify themselves as gay or bisexual," reported Sunny Rumsey. "They identify by their ethnic background. Because they know how their community will respond, they have a tendency to be more closeted about their sexuality." For this reason, C-HAG in Detroit decided not to develop written materials that use labels like Black homosexual, Black gays. Instead, the group designed a poster and brochure describing AIDS as a public health problem that should be of concern to all community members. "By framing the brochure that describes high-risk behavior in more generic terms," explained Linda Williams, "we have attemped to protect the anonymity of individuals who are in need of the information, not fearful of being suspected and labeled as homosexual if they request educational materials or participate in educational encounters."

Deciding how to describe risky sexual practices in a clear yet nonoffensive way is another problem facing AIDS educators in communities of color. "Hispanics have been reluctant to discuss AIDS and sexuality," observed Judy Wenning of New York City's West Side AIDS Project. "Sometimes they consider it rude and insulting. We're working hard to find the right words and ease into it. I think we have to accept some cultural prohibitions." Michele Rigaud, a physician and health educator with Florida's Health Department and the University of Miami, conducted a detailed assessment of sexual practices and values of Cubans, African-Americans, and Haitians living in Florida, and then developed education materials aimed at each group.

The San Francisco focus group of Black, Latino, and Asian leaders strongly believed that most education materials developed by gay AIDS organizations were "too sexually explicit . . . sexual explicitness not only offends readers but also feeds stereotypes about who is at risk for AIDS." The group recommended that "nonmainstream sexual behaviors should be deleted whenever possible." One participant who worked in Asian communities argued, "Face to face, we can use nonverbal expressions and inoffensive signals to communicate about behaviors to be avoided, but when these behaviors are put on the printed page, they cause big problems."

Other educators, however, disagree with this position. Don Edwards, former director of the Spectrum and Alianza AIDS projects in Washington, DC, noted, "Blacks at all levels of their communities know and use the words everyone else uses." He suggested a feedback or focus session with Black people of various backgrounds to get guidance from the specific target population. Edwards also observed that the "best resources" for AIDS education "are the largely overlooked Black people who have been in the fight since the beginning. More are joining every day. In every area in this nation are Black people who can lead in production of the effective educational literature Black communities need so desperately."

Educators must also understand how poverty and discrimination influence people's views of sexuality. "Most Haitians have grown up in a very authoritarian climate," explained Patricia Benoit, an educator with the American Friends Service Committee's Haitian Women's Education Project in New York City. "The government of Haiti controlled most parts of people's lives and when Haitians came to the United States, they encountered racism, unemployment, and legal sanctions. Sex was one of the very few arenas where people could make their own decisions. And so now the same authorities who control the rest of our lives come along and tell us who to have sex with and how to do it. Is it surprising that there is resistance?"

Ruth Rodriguez of the Hispanic AIDS Forum noted that when Latino men were out of work and unable to provide for their families, sex became an even more important element of masculine identity. "Asking the partners of these men to encourage them to wear condoms can be asking for trouble," she said.

Acknowledging cultural differences does not necessarily mean accepting them. Gay men of color have been waging their own battles against homophobia for years, and women of color have developed personal and political strategies for combatting machismo or sexism. "I have no interest in promoting gender roles that teach women they are helpless," said Ruth Rodriguez. Rather, by understanding a population's belief systems, including the contradictory elements in a culture (e.g., the tradition of the strong Black or Latina woman who makes decisions for her family), educators create the possibility for engaging African-American and Latino communities in a dialogue about sexuality and health.

Plan educational interventions that use positive elements of the cultures of African-Americans and Latinos.

Too often, health educators see unfamiliar cultures as an obstacle to be overcome, a barrier to effective education. But some AIDS educators working in Black and Latino communities have adopted a different view, in which culture becomes a vehicle to increase the effectiveness of communication.

Machismo, for example, includes the concept that men are responsible for women and children. Tapping into this belief, rather than personal health protection, may help increase the effectiveness of messages designed to encourage Black and Latino men to use condoms. (At the same time, however, as discussed in Chapter 9, "Women," the double standard for sexual conduct must be challenged by AIDS educators.)

BEBASHI in Philadelphia, Spectrum in Washington, DC, HERO in Baltimore, and other AIDS organizations working in Black and Latino communities have used images of families and children in their AIDS education. The San Francisco focus group on AIDS education recommended that the family theme might also be effective in reaching Latino and Asian populations. "For single Black mothers," observed Annette Johnson of the New York State AIDS Institute, "being sick with AIDS can threaten their self-sufficiency and this might motivate protective action."

Educators working with Haitians in Florida tried another approach to use culture to encourage prevention. An informal meeting between medical AIDS specialists and voodoo folk doctors was arranged to discuss AIDS. At the meeting, held in a Miami coffee shop, the participants explored ways to make sure that both medical and folk practitioners could present accurate information on AIDS without violating either belief system.

"*Confianza,* or trust, is a prerequisite for intimate conversation among Hispanics," said Ruth Rodriguez, "so if I'm going to talk to a Hispanic woman about safer sex, I can't be a distant, impersonal professional. I'm going to talk to her as one woman to another." Adapting "professional standards" to provide for effective communication is an important task for the counselor or educator working in Black and Latino communities.

African-Americans and Latinos have a long history of resistance to oppression and fighting for needed resources. "Many of us in BEBASHI come from a civil rights background," explained Rashidah Hassan, "so we're used to organizing and fighting for what we need." Presenting AIDS as a threat to health and survival opens the door to mobilizing Black and other communities in ways they have mobilized many times before.

Acknowledge the political dimensions of AIDS in African-American and Latino communities.

Dr. Benny Primm, a physician who directs a drug treatment program in Brooklyn, said he is "just about tarred and feathered" when he tells Black audiences that the AIDS virus is not a tool of germ warfare perpetrated by whites.

"Do you think a Black or Hispanic woman is *not* going to think about genocide if I ask her to put off childbearing indefinitely until we do some more research?" incredulously asked a social worker serving drug-using women.

"Most Haitians see AIDS as one more obstacle white America has put into their path to block integration into American society," said Patricia Benoit of the Haitian Women's Education Project.

These quotes illustrate the fact that AIDS cannot be divorced from the social and political context in which Blacks and Latinos live in the United States. Educators who attempt to refute these perceptions face an uphill battle. For one thing, they are deeply rooted in people's personal and collective experience. For another, theories such as the germ warfare genesis of AIDS are almost impossible to disprove (or prove).

Instead, AIDS educators can acknowledge these beliefs, then help a group to decide what to do. "Anger is an important first step," said Annette Johnson, a Black educator with the New York AIDS Institute, "but then people need to take the next step. Educators can play an important role by looking for areas where people can gain control over choices."

A woman considering whether to get pregnant or continue a pregnancy, for example, needs information on HIV transmission rates and the outcome of AIDS in infants. The goal is to help the woman make a choice that she feels is acceptable. When it is emphasized that the decision is hers, the feeling that a professional—often a white professional—is imposing his or her choice is reduced.

For those working with Haitians, acknowledging the political dimensions means that one cannot discuss HIV antibody testing without looking at the purpose to which the results may be put. If the result of being tested is to lose the opportunity to attain legal status in the United States, educators must present this possibility clearly.

Use community institutions to reach African-American and Latino populations.

"Look at who is already doing education in your community," advised Rashidah Hassan, "and get them to add AIDS to their agenda." For BEBASHI, as described in

Chapter 3, this meant working with churches, tenant organizations, elected officials, and the local chapter of the NAACP. Another group in Philadelphia, the Philadelphia AIDS Task Force, developed a curriculum designed to teach ministers how to integrate AIDS education into their pastoral responsibilities.

Nashville CARES helped churches and Black health professionals disseminate information on AIDS. C-HAG in Detroit runs "rap shops," informal seminars on AIDS for local community groups. Specific methods for helping neighborhood organizations take on AIDS are described in the "Community Education" section in Chapter 4.

As AIDS becomes a growing issue in African-American and Latino communities, more and more community organizations will be willing to play a role in prevention. AIDS educators face no more important challenge than empowering community organizations to meet the threat of HIV infection.

C H A P T E R   E I G H T

Youth

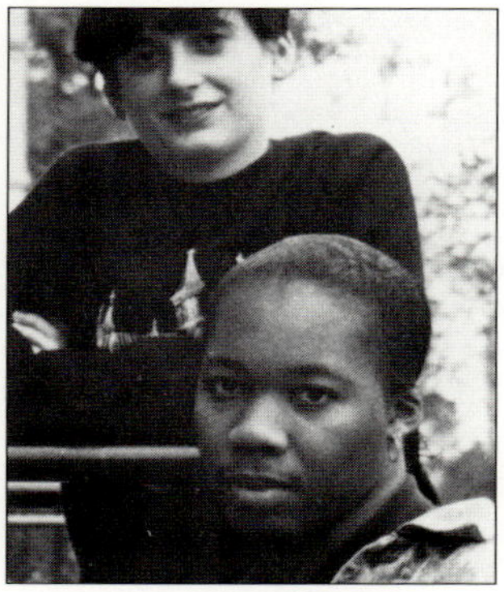

CASE HISTORY

*Teens Rap About Drugs, STDs, and AIDS, San Francisco**

"Rap" is an ideal vehicle to carry messages about AIDS prevention because it is an accepted part of teen culture, as well as a highly political art form. The term "rap" encompasses a number of speech forms common in Black vernacular English. The term is currently used to refer to a popular form of spontaneous rhyming with a structured rhythmic base that is common among Black and Latino teenagers in the urban inner city.

San Francisco health educators, representing the Bayview-Hunter's Point Foundation and the city department of public health, recently used a rap contest to reach teenagers—and to enable them to reach each other—with AIDS prevention information. Fifty San Francisco teenagers competed in a city-wide rap contest on the theme "Rapn' Down Drugs, STDs and AIDS." Preliminary rounds of the contest were held in local youth centers throughout the city, and the final round was taped

* This case history is an edited version of an article about a citywide "rap" contest, from the newsletter *Multicultural Inquiry and Research on AIDS,* spring 1987. It was written by Mindy Fullilove, MD. The raps quoted are reproduced exactly as they appeared in the young people's original submissions to the contest.

and shown on the popular local television show, "Home Turf."

Raps, which were judged for content as well as the performer's style and delivery, demonstrated a strong concern with AIDS: as one young author wrote, "AIDS Is Destroying Society." They had vivid images of AIDS as a new, deadly disease but one that could be prevented, as these lines show:

Before you lay down for a love connection
you better make sure you have protection
If you wind up with the thing they call aids
It just may leave you laying in your grave.

The rappers focused on the damage that drugs were doing, both directly and as a way of transmitting AIDS. In "Drugs are on the Rise," the rapper commented:

Drugs in your bank account will leave
a big dent After your money is spent
you'll just resent
Feel as IF you Just lost your best friend,
so In order to mend
You'll go and get some more again, But
the only thing your doing is
Living in Peril, First class ticket to hell
as your refferel,
The best way out is Just to avoid or
you'll get No sleep,
Never eat
Worry be PArANoid. You could lose close,
home, gold, even pounds, so leave drugs
alone that's all I'm trying to announce.

The rappers depicted the plight of the addict with a combination of understanding and impatience: "Stop using drug and use your head, before you O.D. and wind up dead."

The rappers uniformly urged sex with precautions such as condoms and limiting the number of sexual partners, but none expressed disapproval of premarital sex. Marcus, in "STDs and AIDS," rapped:

I'm here to talk about the S in STD
because the S stands for sexually
And to the right of S the T is committed
for the simple reason T is transmitted.
So if I may please, especially with ease,
freeze,
and tell you that the D stands for
disease
So you better watch out if you know
what I mean,
don't take a floosey, be choosey and
you'll stay clean.

More information about the rappers was obtained by pretest and posttest administrations of the AIDS Literacy Test, a 10-item scale developed to assess knowledge of basic facts about AIDS. Rappers had a mean score of 9 out of 10, with no significant difference on the pretest and posttest administrations. Thus, despite their lack of educational achievements, this group of young people was at least minimally informed about AIDS, including the major methods of transmission and the options for protection. The young people were aware of the high-risk groups, and they were aware of the dangers to Blacks and Latinos, as well as to heterosexuals.

"Rapn' Down Drugs, STDs and AIDS" involved San Francisco minority teenagers in AIDS prevention. The raps have become public service announcements that can be heard on San Francisco radio stations, thus reaching a far wider audience. This model of prevention education can be used to reach Black and Latino youth throughout the United States. Adult support of this prevention strategy can effectively mobilize teenagers to act to decrease their risk for AIDS.

CASE HISTORY

Covenant House, New York City

A few blocks from Times Square and down the street from the Port Authority Bus Terminal, in the heart of New York City's sex industry district, Covenant House provides crisis care—food, shelter, clothing, medical treatment, and job counseling—for homeless youth. Two years ago, Covenant House also added AIDS education to its mission.

In 1987, 28 teenagers seen in the Covenant House's health clinic tested positive for HIV. An anonymous serosurvey released in 1988 showed that 4% of the sample of homeless youth tested were infected with HIV. "What we see now in terms of cases is only the tip of the iceberg," noted Ann Donahue, director of the off-the-street outreach program. "The kids are out there getting sick now, and we will see them become sicker over the next few years."

Father Bruce Ritter, director of Covenant House, attributes the high risk of HIV infection to prostitution—"their selling and our buying of sex." Other staff members report that residents frequently use drugs, especially crack, and often in exchange for sex. Homeless youth are particularly vulnerable to HIV infection. "Living on the streets, the kids are exposed to everything," said Donahue. "They turn to drugs very quickly. They are very lonely, and it's a way to escape the reality of the streets." She went on to explain that "kids who are out on the streets don't take precautions. They don't think they are going to die anyway. Contracting AIDS is the least worry on their mind."

To address this situation, Covenant House AIDS educator Joan Altman developed a program that would provide young people with the information and skills that could protect them. Since 1987, she has been leading daily sessions on AIDS for residents of the shelter. Altman begins her session by giving out snacks. "So many of these kids don't eat, so food helps them to stay awake," she notes. A film provides some basic facts on AIDS. Although a few viewers snort with derision when the film advocates abstinence, most watch attentively. When it is over, they pepper Altman with questions. "I just check if a girl is clean before I go with her," says one young man, "so I don't need to worry, right?" "Wrong," replies Altman. "There's no way to tell if someone has the disease by looking at them. You could take ten showers a day and still be infected." With humor, patience, and respect, Altman elicits and corrects the misinformation that circulates on the streets.

Altman also provides one-to-one counseling to young people who are perceived to be at risk of HIV infection. She provides information, assesses concerns, and makes referrals as necessary. She also leads staff training sessions that focus on panic reduction "so that when we have a resident known to be HIV-positive or with ARC or AIDS, staff members know they have nothing to fear." She also helps staff work out their feelings about homosexuality, stressing Covenant House's pledge to serve kids with "unconditional love and acceptance" and provide sanctuary with no judgment.

Because Covenant House is a Catholic agency, it does not distribute condoms. Other agencies serving the homeless youth of the Times Square area do, however, provide condoms, making them relatively accessible to street youth.

Father Ritter announces proudly that Covenant House "never turns a kid away. We provide the kind of help these kids need when they come here and there's no other place to go." To fulfill this pledge, Covenant House is now opening a residence for teenagers with AIDS and ARC, the first such facility of its kind, and a grim reminder of the impact of the epidemic on New York City's youth.

CASE HISTORY

American Red Cross AIDS Prevention Program for Youth

The American Red Cross AIDS Prevention Program for Youth seeks to provide youth of junior and senior high school age with the information, education materials, and training needed to choose behaviors that reduce their risk of contracting HIV infection. According to Carole Kaufman, manager of the American Red Cross AIDS education program, its youth services are "a community- and family-based program."

To develop a film aimed at Black and Latino youth, the Red Cross worked with a network of family planning providers in Chicago. A script for the film was market tested in nine cities with teens, parents, youth-serving agencies, and community leaders. Based on suggestions from these panels, the film's message on drugs was made more hard hitting.

In the production, "Don't Forget Sherrie," a group of Black teens learn that a former girlfriend, Sherrie, is dying of AIDS, possibly contracted while sharing needles with other IV drug users. The Chicago school system and the Chicago Urban League both played a role in making the film.

The Red Cross youth program seeks to—

- increase educators' acceptance of the need for AIDS education in the schools;
- increase teachers' ability to provide AIDS education;
- increase parents' ability to discuss AIDS with their children;
- reach adolescents who are not part of the school program.

To ensure that its materials do not offend its supporters, the Red Cross program emphasizes to youth that "they can avoid contracting AIDS by saying 'no' to sex and 'no' to drugs." The American Red Cross AIDS Prevention Program for Youth demonstrates how a national organization can contribute to the development of comprehensive community-based AIDS education aimed at young people.

A Rationale for AIDS Education for Young People

For no other group are the benefits of AIDS prevention more clear-cut than for children and young people. On the one hand, the prevalence of HIV infection and AIDS in this age group is extremely low, and, on the other hand, the behaviors that put young people in the path of HIV are alarmingly widespread. These two factors, combined with the social and economic advantages of intervening *before* risky behaviors become well established, make AIDS education for young people a high priority. This chapter focuses on AIDS education for young people aged 12 to 21. Most experts agree that sex education should begin in the primary school years and that in terms of AIDS, the principal goal is to establish a foundation for more specific learning in later years. A detailed discussion of the content and methods of sex education for younger children is beyond the scope of this guide. Interested readers should consult the "Resources" section for useful references.

According to the Centers for Disease Control, only 336 cases of AIDS had been diagnosed in those aged 13 to 19 as of late 1988, less than 1% of all cases. Adolescents between 13 and 19 comprise about 10% of the American population, or about 25 million individuals. A variety of surveys of HIV prevalence also show very low rates among adolescents. For example, among New York City applicants for military service under the age of 18 during the 1985-86 period, HIV seroprevalence was 0.23%. For 18- to 21-year-olds, the seroprevalence was 0.31%. For applicants 25 or older, seroprevalence was nearly 13 times higher than for those under 18. Despite these low numbers, however, health programs serving young people in urban areas report increasing encounters with HIV-infected teenagers. And as mentioned previously, a New York City serosurvey of homeless youth showed a significant level of HIV infection in 1988.

A review of data on young people's sexual and drug behavior provides additional cause for concern. About half of all adolescents have had sexual intercourse by the age of 19. For urban and nonwhite adolescents, first intercourse tends to be at younger ages. According to one study of girls in detention centers in the Bronx, the average age of first intercourse was 12. Nationally, 16% of teenage women report having had four or more sexual partners. Each year in the United States there are 1.2 million pregnancies among teenage girls. Health officials estimate that one in seven teenagers currently has a sexually transmitted disease. About half of sexually experienced adolescents use contraception at first intercourse, one-third to one-fourth have never used contraception, and only about 12% of teenagers report using condoms. Data on the prevalence of homosexual activity among teens are lacking. One study in the mid-1970s found that 17% of boys aged 16 to 19 reported at least one homosexual experience. More recent studies show higher rates. What proportion of those with homosexual experience in adolescence go on to define themselves as gay or bisexual is unknown.

Drug experts estimate conservatively that more than 200,000 high school students have used heroin. Millions of others have tried cocaine, stimulants, or other opiates, all of which can be injected intravenously. Drug use is much higher among high school dropouts. In some urban African-American and Latino communities, school dropout rates exceed 50%. Few drug treatment programs are equipped to serve adolescents. In New York City, for example, most programs will not accept teenage addicts. The epidemic of crack use in certain urban areas in the past three years has created a pattern of behavior particularly conducive to the spread of HIV infection, as described in Chapter 6, "Intravenous Drug Users."

At highest risk of HIV infection are the growing population of teenagers who are homeless, engaging in prostitution, using drugs, and often receiving inadequate health and social services. It is estimated that 1 million minors run away from home every year and that between 125,000 and 200,000 male and female teenagers engage in prostitution. Most runaways are not the stereotypical white middle-class girls from the suburban Midwest, but rather urban Black or Latino youth. In New York City alone, advocacy groups estimate that at least 10,000 young people do not have a home.

Some of the developmental characteristics of teenagers also have implications for their receptivity to AIDS education. For many, the adolescent years are a time to assert independence from authority figures and parents. This normal healthy process can lead teens to question the reliability or relevance of AIDS messages, particularly if they are presented in a moralistic fashion.

Conversely, the role of the peer group is strong. When peer values support sexual and drug experimentation, a young person may have difficulty in making a decision to abstain.

Young people may also believe themselves invulnerable to serious illness. "When I was an adolescent," reported an AIDS educator in San Francisco, "I thought I knew everything. Nobody could tell me anything. Nothing was going to touch me or harm me. I was definitely smarter than any adult I knew. The kids we work with feel the same way, and somehow we need to understand that."

Adolescence is also a time of experimentation. Young people seek to define for themselves values, roles, and behaviors that seem right. In some cases, such experimentation can cause troubling but manageable conflicts with parents or other adults; in other cases it can lead to serious harm, even death. The use of alcohol or other drugs increases the likelihood of taking dangerous risks.

What Young People Know About AIDS

A review of several surveys of young people's knowledge and attitudes about AIDS reveals the following generalizations:

- Most teenagers (80% to 90%) know that AIDS is spread through sexual intercourse and use of IV drugs. Fewer know the specific fluids believed to carry the virus.
- A smaller majority (60% to 70%) know specific methods of protection against transmission, including use of condoms and cleaning of needles.
- A significant minority of teenagers believe that AIDS can be caught from donating blood or from nonsexual contact with an infected person.
- Black and Latino young people are somewhat less likely to have accurate knowledge and considerably more likely to fear catching AIDS through nonsexual contact.
- Television and newspapers are the primary source of AIDS information for young people.
- According to a 1987 random sample of Massachusetts youth aged 16 to 19, 15% of those who were sexually active reported changing their sexual behavior because of concern about AIDS. Of these, 10% reported use of condoms and 35% reported that they were more selective of their partners, a strategy unlikely to adequately protect them.

What these data show is that although most young people have some accurate information about AIDS, more specific information is needed to enable young people to protect themselves. A suggested list of messages for young people is provided in Figure 28. More important, survey findings show clearly that information is not sufficient to change behavior. AIDS educators working with young people will need strategies that help learners use information in acting to prevent the spread of HIV infection.

Debra Haffner of the Center for Population Options, a Washington, D.C., research and policy institute concerned with adolescent reproduction and health, suggested the following four goals for AIDS prevention programs for adolescents:

- Reduce the panic and misinformation about the disease and its transmission.
- Help teenagers delay the initiation of sexual intercourse.
- Ensure that teenagers who are having any type of intercourse use condoms consistently and effectively.
- Reduce experimentation with drugs and prevent HIV drug use.

Figure 28. WHAT YOUNG PEOPLE SHOULD KNOW ABOUT AIDS*

AIDS is a disease caused by a virus that prevents the body from fighting off certain diseases that healthy people usually do not catch. AIDS is usually fatal.

People catch AIDS in three main ways:

- Through getting infected blood inside their body by sharing needles, syringes, or works used to inject drugs;
- Through infected semen and vaginal fluid that gets inside the partner's body through anal, vaginal, or oral sex;
- Inside a mother's uterus if the mother is infected with the virus.

Anyone who engages in risky behaviors can become infected, whether they are male or female, gay or straight, young or old, white, Black, Latino, or Asian.

People do not catch the virus that causes AIDS by hugging, sneezing, sharing bathrooms, or swimming in a pool. It is a hard disease to get.

Some people contracted AIDS by getting a transfusion of blood infected with the virus. Now, however, all blood is tested and the blood supply is extremely safe. There is *no* danger of getting AIDS by *donating* blood.

People who are infected with the virus—

- May have no symptoms of disease. Because they look and feel healthy, they may not know they are infected. They can pass on the virus to other people in the three ways described earlier. Many of these people will eventually get sick, but some may be healthy for several years after they have first become infected.
- Some who are infected may have symptoms related to AIDS, such as swollen glands or serious infections, but not be officially counted as cases of AIDS. They may be mildly ill or very sick.
- May have the disease AIDS, for which at present there is no cure. Many medicines do, however, control the infections that people with AIDS catch.

Testing

It is now possible to test a person's blood to see if that person has been exposed to the virus that causes AIDS. The test does *not* tell if the person has AIDS. At present, public health officials do not recommend the test for most teenagers. Young people who have engaged in risky behavior, especially those who are pregnant or considering pregnancy (having a baby or fathering a baby), should discuss the test with a doctor.

Young people can prevent getting infected with HIV by:

- Not having sex.
- Always using condoms (even in combination with other methods of birth control such as the pill) from beginning to end of oral, anal, or vaginal sexual intercourse.
- Not using IV drugs. Those who do should not share needles, syringes, or works. Tattoo needles or needles for another drug should never be shared.

For more information

Young people should get information on local and national sources of AIDS information, including telephone hotlines.

---

* Based on materials prepared by the National Coalition of Advocates for Students.

Settings for Educating Young People About AIDS

Whenever young people congregate, AIDS educators need to establish programs. By making prevention messages pervasive, our society begins to create a climate that ensures that all young people know how to protect themselves and are able to take action to prevent the spread of HIV infection.

Schools

Schools reach more young people than any other institution. Their stated mission is to educate children and youth, and thus they become a logical focus for AIDS education. By early 1987, according to a survey by the US Conference of Mayors, 54% of 73 of the largest school districts already offered some form of AIDS education to high school students. Many others were considering establishing requirements. In the past two years, state education departments throughout the nation have been developing curriculum guidelines for AIDS education.

The following questions address some of the issues those planning school-based AIDS education programs need to consider.

Who should plan the curriculum for AIDS education programs? In most areas, the state education department sets curriculum and local school boards, superintendents, and teachers implement it to fit local conditions. Inevitably, the process is political. When a subject is as controversial as AIDS, involving sex, drugs, and death, political factors can become decisive.

Astute AIDS educators can prevent political problems by involving concerned parties early in the planning process. They also increase these groups' stakes in the program, and they create an opportunity to educate community leaders as well as children.

Some advocate letting local school boards decide on AIDS education. Former Secretary of Health and Human Services Otis Bowen argued, "The way out is . . . to let each community decide for itself. Local school boards are excellent sounding boards for community attitudes, so it is both right and reasonable to let them decide."

One problem with this approach is that in those districts where the school board does not reflect the larger community, a small group of people may make decisions that are unpopular with significant portions of the population. Moreover, assigning responsibility to local school boards absolves state agencies of their responsibility to provide funding, model curriculums, technical assistance, and training. At best, however, a partnership between local school boards and state education departments can lead to a program that is pedagogically sound and politically acceptable.

Another approach is to establish an external advisory or planning committee to work with sex educators and school officials at the local level to plan new curriculums or to advise on implementation of an existing one. Such committees can include mental health, child health, and public health professionals; clergy (both liberal and conservative); parents; teachers; students; and others.

Mary Lee Tatum, coordinator of the Falls Church, VA, school sex education and family living program, advised against including in such a committee fundamentalist or conservative groups that are inalterably opposed to any sex education in the schools. "If you were going to prepare an English curriculum, would you include someone who didn't believe we should teach English in the schools?" she asked. Once such a planning group is recruited, its members must receive training on the dimensions of the problem. "Don't assume that this astute group of people you have brought together knows what needs to be done," warned Tatum. "Spend two or three sessions educating them about AIDS and sex education."

Tatum suggested that groups seeking to bring AIDS education into the school approach parent/teacher associations and school boards first. "Don't go to administrators" she said, "because they don't have the power. School boards and parents do." She also recommended approaching ministerial associations rather than individual churches, because these associations reflect broader cross-sections of the community and more diverse ideological perspectives.

By enlisting a variety of constituencies in planning AIDS education, planners create sufficient political support for a program to defend against attacks by conservative or religious groups. Public opinion polls show that most parents support school sex education. Surveys of parents in San Francisco showed that only 20 out of 22,000 parents removed their children from AIDS education classes; less than 1% of Denver parents did not want their children to attend AIDS education classes. A 1987 NBC national poll found that 91% of adults approved of teaching AIDS prevention in public schools. Effective AIDS educators mobilize these majorities to support their work.

How should AIDS education be connected to the larger curriculum? Most AIDS educators agree that one or two sessions on AIDS are probably not sufficient to provide young people with adequate information, much less to teach relevant decision-making skills. In the crisis mentality that often sweeps over public officials, however, new problems facing young people are often assigned no more than a few hours of class time. Although this approach is not desirable, in some locations it may be all that is possible, and AIDS educators should seek to ensure that these few sessions address real concerns and that they refer young people to other sources of information and services. In some cases, successful short-term programs can lay the groundwork for more comprehensive plans.

Educators have proposed a variety of strategies for linking information on AIDS to other subjects in the school curriculum. Stephan Sroka, a classroom teacher and author of the *Educator's Guide to AIDS and Other STDs,* strongly believes that information on AIDS should (a) be presented in an overall conceptual framework focusing on communicable diseases and (b) stress a behavioral approach to prevention strategies.

One rationale for looking at AIDS as a communicable disease is that few are opposed to discussing disease prevention in the schools. Putting AIDS in a more clinical perspective can defuse some of the opposition and anxiety that the subject can arouse in parents, teachers, and students. On the other hand, such an approach can make it easier to avoid altogether the discussions about sex, drugs, and relationships that young people need to have. In an extreme example of this danger, a health department official responsible for planning AIDS education in schools in a Midwestern city reported, "I don't talk about sex, I talk about viruses and how they are transmitted."

Most AIDS educators believe that the most logical place for AIDS teaching is in sex education and family living curriculums. "After all, AIDS is part and parcel of sex education," said Mary Lee Tatum. "What we need to teach is a decision-making process." Where a sex education curriculum is already in place, the foundation for AIDS education—male and female anatomy and physiology, sexual values, STDs, relationships, contraception, homosexuality—has already been constructed.

Adding sessions on AIDS then becomes a relatively simple task. Moreover, experienced sex education teachers may already have some of the skills and information needed to cover this subject, reducing the need for additional training.

For those committed to maintaining a positive view of human sexuality, sex education provides a context for explaining the risks of AIDS without moralizing or instilling inappropriate fears. "The goal of sexuality education," said Michael Carrera, a prominent sex educator, "is to give young people the dual message that sexuality is a positive life force, a gift, and that people need to make informed decisions about how to use that force in a way that keeps them healthy."

Where sex education is part of a broader health education curriculum, it makes sense to include AIDS issues in that larger framework. Many such curriculums now emphasize decision-making skills that help young people avoid cigarettes, alcohol, illegal drugs, dangerous driving, and STDs.

Still another approach is to integrate AIDS education with other academic subjects. According to Jonathan Silin, director of education for the Long Island Association for AIDS Care: "AIDS education should not be the sole province of the health teacher. In civics classes, it might be appropriate in an election year to involve students in discussions of the candidates' position on AIDS. Biology classes could be an appropriate forum to introduce basic concepts in epidemiology." By addressing AIDS from a variety of perspectives, it is possible to prepare young people for the individual and collective tasks that the AIDS epidemic will impose on them in the years to come. Figure 29 provides a checklist developed by the National Coalition of Advocates for Students to assess AIDS education curricula. The Centers for Disease Control has also issued guidelines for school AIDS curriculums.

Figure 29. CHECKLIST FOR EVALUATING AIDS CURRICULUMS*

Curriculum Content

- Does the curriculum give simple, clear, and direct information? Is that information given in terms, including slang, that students understand? (See Figure 30 for content of information.)
- Does the curriculum focus on teaching healthy behaviors and not just on the biomedical aspects of the disease?
- By emphasizing high-risk behaviors rather than high-risk groups, does the curriculum strongly convey the message that anyone can get AIDS regardless of race, sex, age, or sexual orientation?
- Are several class periods provided to give students multiple opportunities to learn to make decisions based on the information they have learned about AIDS?

Development and Implementation

- Does the program provide for adequate training to teach the curriculum?
- Is the same information made available to limited English proficient students in their own language? Is the information provided appropriately to hearing-impaired and visually impaired students and students with severely handicapping conditions?
- Is the curriculum updated regularly to incorporate new information as it becomes available?
- Has the curriculum been developed with the participation and support of parents, students, and other community groups? Does it facilitate an ongoing dialogue with parents on these issues?

* Based on materials developed by the National Coalition of Advocates for Students.

What else can schools do to encourage AIDS prevention? A carefully conceived curriculum on AIDS education is a necessary part of a school-based AIDS prevention program, but educational institutions can do much more. The following examples illustrate how the school can become a focal point for other interventions:

- In a high school in New York City, AIDS educators trained a group of students to become peer AIDS educators. These peer educators provided their schoolmates with accurate information and referrals related to AIDS in informal settings such as the cafeteria or after school hours.
- San Francisco's school AIDS education program offers high school students physical exams in their schools' "teen clinics" if they request them. Students are also provided information on HIV antibody testing.
- A special issue of LASSO, the student newspaper of the George Mason Junior/Senior High School in Falls Church, VA, was devoted to AIDS; student reporters interviewed scientists, public health officials, and people with AIDS.
- The Cincinnati Board of Education instituted a family life and sex education curriculum for kindergarten through 12th grade that includes special training for teachers at a nearby university.
- The New York City Board of Education is training "parent trainers" to conduct parent workshops on AIDS in the public schools. It has also trained outreach staff of settlement houses to provide AIDS education services to out-of-school youth, a population usually neglected by school-based programs.
- The Maryland AIDS Foundation in Rockville, MD, recruited volunteers for its Teen AIDS Hotline at high school assembly presentations on AIDS.

By planning programs for each constituency that they interact with (students, parents, teachers, staff, administrators, truants), schools can help create a climate in which prevention can become a priority. Furthermore, each group that is educated can reinforce messages for the other group. For example, many parents report that school programs help children to educate their parents about AIDS.

Should controversial subjects be discussed? No aspect of the AIDS epidemic has generated more controversy than what to teach young people. There is much debate over whether school-based AIDS education programs should discuss controversial subjects such as safer sex, condom use, homosexuality, and how to sterilize drug equipment. Conservatives like Senator Jesse Helms and Phyllis Schlafly argue that much AIDS education teaches "safer sodomy" and that it is "a violation of the First Amendment rights of children whose religion teaches that nonmarital sexual acts are wrong." While he was secretary of education, William J. Bennett wrote in a handbook on AIDS distributed in 1987 by the US Department of Education that "young people should be told that the best way to prevent the sexual transmission of AIDS is to refrain from sexual activity until as adults they are ready to establish a mutually faithful monogamous relationship." He also wrote that "materials discussing illicit drugs should not condone 'responsible use' or use of 'soft drugs'. All illicit drug use is wrong."

Others reject such a moralistic tone, for both public health and pedagogical reasons. New York City Health Commissioner Stephen Joseph argued that high schools should give sexually active young people "access to condoms, which will protect them." Similarly, Surgeon General C. Everett Koop has said that for the 70% of adolescents who are already sexually active, "you have to introduce condoms, knowing that it offends the sensitivities of some people."

Mary Lee Tatum, sex education coordinator, raised another objection. "When was the last time you asked an adolescent to do something and they did it? . . . From a pedagogical point of view," she explained, "the 'just say no' campaign ignores what we know about adolescent development." She suggested instead presenting young people with what we know about AIDS, outlining the strategies for protection including both abstinence and safer sex, and then saying, "You need to decide for yourselves what you want from life and how you are going to protect yourself against this terrible disease." Such an approach does not preclude adults from explaining their own moral views.

Although a broad-based planning committee will help devise a politically acceptable approach to sensitive topics, in many communities it is unlikely that any process will guarantee a solution that satisfies everybody. Experienced sex educators suggest the following strategies for teaching controversial subjects:

- Educate all relevant constituencies *before* the program begins. Explain your goals and rationale clearly and forthrightly.
- Organize and mobilize constituencies that will support your programs.
- Emphasize that school programs are not a substitute for a parental role in sex education. Parents have the right to transmit their values to their children. Schools also have the responsibility to provide young people with information and skills they can use to protect their health and the health of others.
- Discuss the role of the community in public health. Preventing the further spread of HIV infection requires community as well as individual action. When a community disagrees about how to proceed, in a democratic society the majority rules, barring violation of fundamental rights. In our legal system, there are clear prohibitions against any religious group's using public schools to advance a particular viewpoint. There are no constitutional barriers against providing health or sex education.
- Planners should keep sight of their long-term goals. Developing and implementing a curriculum that is less than ideal, but politically acceptable, may be more desirable than a more explicit approach that will serve as a rallying point for opponents. Partial victories can pave the way for more profound changes over time.

Colleges and Universities

About 12 million students, or 5% of the nation's adult population, are enrolled in institutions of higher learning in the United States. Because the college years are often a time for experimentation with sex and drugs, young people attending colleges and universities are in great need of education about AIDS. Moreover, the period between high school and full-time work and family responsibilities often provides young people with an opportunity to consider their attitudes, values, and lifestyles more carefully than during other life stages. Positive behaviors established then can influence health throughout life. And as Cathy Kodama, coordinator of the AIDS education program at the University of California at Berkeley, noted: "The campus is readily suited for public health interventions. The student community is a definable population existing in a 'contained,' accessible environment. The adoption of educational campaigns is facilitated by existing systems for community organization, policy development, and instruction."

In urban areas with a high prevalence of HIV infection, universities and community colleges with large enrollments of African-American and Latino youth provide good forums for reaching young people at higher risk of AIDS. College students are also potentially effective community and family health educators.

AIDS educators working on college campuses have used a variety of methods to get AIDS prevention messages out. Most of these use techniques described in earlier chapters of this guide, adapted to the particular characteristics of the college setting.

Peer education. Before the AIDS epidemic, many colleges offered training to interested students so that they could provide their peers with accurate information and referrals about contraception, sexuality, alcohol, drugs, and other health topics. AIDS became one more issue for peer educators to address. At Dartmouth College in New Hampshire, for example, peer educators lead informal dormitory discussions on abstinence, contraception, and STDs. Because small group discussions have been demonstrated to be an effective way to help people change health behaviors, this model is well suited to AIDS education. Peer educators also become advocates for AIDS prevention policies and programs in the college community.

Another approach to peer education is to use resident assistants or advisors to provide information. In fall 1987, the American College Health Association and Gay Men's Health Crisis offered training for students working in college dormitories throughout New York City. Participants learned how to answer questions, make referrals, and involve students in discussions of drugs and sex.

Planners of peer education programs must consider how to recruit volunteers, how much training to provide, and how to supervise peer educators. See the "Training" section in Chapter 4 for more information.

Special events. In October 1986, during its annual Health Week, New York University sponsored "A Discussion on AIDS: Current Topics on Treatment and Prevention." Prominent scientists and clinicians spoke to more than 600 attendees.

San Francisco Community College sponsored an AIDS Awareness Week in February 1986 that included panel discussions, safer-sex workshops, films, plays, and exhibits. Some regularly scheduled classes featured invited speakers on AIDS during the week.

Events such as these provide opportunities to provide information, distribute education materials, provoke discussion, and raise awareness of the AIDS issue. They also enable AIDS activists to identify and recruit other students and faculty who can become involved in future AIDS prevention activities.

College health services. College health services provide an excellent forum for AIDS education. At Rutgers University in New Jersey, for example, the AIDS epidemic prompted the student health service to mandate that clinicians provide *all* students with an STD education packet. This included information on gonorrhea, syphilis, chlamydia, AIDS, and other STDs, and a condom. Clinicians explain that these materials are provided to all students regardless of the reason for the clinic visit. Students are asked if they have any questions and are told of other resources such as health counseling, education programs, and psychological services.

Other health services provide AIDS counseling and education, AIDS literature, mental health services, and referrals for drug treatment. A few offer HIV antibody testing. Barnard College in New York City, for instance, decided that a campus-based testing program could counsel its students more sensitively and appropriately than off-campus test sites. Colleges that consider offering HIV testing must address the issues of confidentiality, support and referrals for HIV-positive students, and the adequacy of resources for pretest and posttest counseling.

An AIDS educator at a college in Philadelphia that offered HIV testing warned that for many college students, the test is a quick fix for concerns about exposure. "We have lots of students who come in saying, 'I had sex with someone new on Friday night, so give me the AIDS test.' " These students often refuse or resist counseling and "in my opinion," the educator said, "having the test available right here is a distraction from the real education that needs to happen."

Development of university policies and programs. The American College Health Association's Task Force on AIDS has urged colleges and universities to develop policies or guidelines to address the range of issues that the AIDS epidemic raises. Waiting until a crisis unfolds makes the task of deciding an appropriate response much more difficult. National organizations, local AIDS groups, and student organizations, particularly gay student groups, have all worked to encourage rational policies on AIDS.

An important first step is to ensure that the leaders of an institution understand the dimensions of the epidemic. At American University in Washington, DC, the top management, a total of 54 persons, attended a 2½-hour session on AIDS epidemiology and policy issues. Mid-level managers participated in a shorter session. These seminars helped the university leadership understand and support subsequent education programs for faculty and students.

On a national level, the American College Health Association established a task force on AIDS, issued a publication on AIDS and the college campus, and prepared policy statements on dormitory issues, confidentiality, athletic competition, and clinical issues for college health services. These guides provide individual colleges with a framework for developing institutional policies.

Many colleges have established AIDS task forces that include administrators, faculty, staff, and students. Such groups can help develop or recommend policies that acknowledge the concerns and needs of various constituencies.

Condom campaigns. Making condoms more readily available and more acceptable to students is an important goal of many college AIDS programs. At the University of Vermont in Burlington, the student newspaper inserted a free condom and a "safer-sex packet" in 5,000 copies of a special issue on AIDS. The issue disappeared swiftly and provoked many discussions on campus.

At New York University, the AIDS education committee arranged to have a condom machine installed in the laundry room of a dormitory. Condom dispensers are also in the male and female bathrooms at the student center. Such efforts serve to make condoms more acceptable and visible. To that end, an AIDS group at the State University of New York (SUNY) at Stony Brook sponsored a contest in a dormitory asking students to guess the number of condoms in a fish bowl. At Hunter College in New York City, AIDS educators distributed "goody bags" with condoms and chocolate kisses on Halloween.

While many college students continue to resist using condoms, others are changing their attitudes. Richard Keeling, director of the student health services at the University of Virginia, reported that many young women now ask him "if it's recommended that they carry condoms in their purse on a date." Only a few years ago, he noted, "such concerns would've gotten laughed out of the room."

Curriculum. Still another approach to campus education is to offer courses on AIDS. SUNY at Stony Brook has developed an AIDS curriculum for colleges and trained educators at more than 50 SUNY campuses in how to use it. Topics covered include facts about AIDS, AIDS and sexuality, AIDS and substance abuse, ethical issues and AIDS, and decision making and AIDS. The curriculum was prepared so that it can be presented as a 15-hour seminar for academic credit, a 6-hour workshop, or a 2-hour instructional program.

Other colleges have integrated AIDS topics into health education, biology, ethics, sociology, and other courses. At Hunter College, for example, one semester of a regularly scheduled course called "Controversial Issues in Health" was devoted entirely to AIDS. AIDS organizations can offer college faculty training programs designed to help them integrate AIDS topics into their curriculum.

Youth Programs

A variety of organizations offer programs for young people: recreation centers, Boys and Girls Clubs, Boy Scouts and Girl Scouts, 4-H Clubs, churches and synagogues, and community centers. It is estimated that youth agencies serve 20 million young people each year. They are an excellent vehicle for reaching adolescents and their parents, for mobilizing volunteers, and for providing credible information in a nonacademic setting. Many such programs also serve out-of-school youth, a population in great need of AIDS education. Because youth agencies often have a history of providing health and sex education, adding AIDS prevention to their mission may not encounter strong opposition.

Three examples of AIDS programs presented by youth agencies follow.

First, the Pilsen Catholic Youth Center in Chicago's Latino community is training young people aged 16 to 21 to be AIDS peer educators in their own neighborhood; it also runs safer-sex talks for teens and parents and sponsors community forums on AIDS for young people.

Second, a comprehensive program for teens in Central Harlem in New York City, run by the Children's Aid Society in a public housing project, provides health services, tutoring, employment, sports, theater, and family life and sex education. In 15 weekly two-hour sessions, teenagers and parents are taught how to integrate sexuality into the rest of their lives. One of the topics covered is AIDS, but the course as a whole emphasizes informed decision making.

Third, the Institute for the Protection of Gay and Lesbian Youth in New York City runs AIDS education programs in a recreation center and in a storefront near the downtown piers and warehouses where prostitution flourishes. Street workers provide counseling and distribute condoms. They also sponsor support groups for young people who need additional help.

In order to develop effective programs, youth agencies need help from AIDS organizations. AIDS educators can provide staff training, appropriate education materials, and technical assistance on program development and implementation. The goal is to help youth agencies acquire the skills and resources needed to integrate ongoing AIDS prevention activities into their existing mission. For additional suggestions, see the "Community Education" section in Chapter 4.

These are suggestions for effective integration of AIDS prevention into existing youth organizations:

- Involve staff and young people in defining goals and content of AIDS prevention activities.
- Link AIDS issues with existing concerns of the youth agency, such as drug abuse prevention, teenage pregnancy, rights of African-Americans and Latinos, and community improvement. "When you start to talk to young people about AIDS," said Curtis Wadlington of Blacks Educating Blacks About Sexual Health Issues in Philadelphia, "you end up talking about relationships, school, stress, being yourself, physical and mental health, caring about other people."
- Look for many ways to engage young people in AIDS prevention; one cannot give a message once and expect people to get it.
- Acknowledge and include positive elements of youth culture such as trust among friends, desire for independence, and dislike of hypocrisy.
- Use the energy and enthusiasm of young people themselves to create momentum for education.
- Give agencies and young people time to grapple with the issue and their concerns; don't expect immediate results or interest.

Health Care Settings

Health care settings provide additional opportunities to educate young people about AIDS. Family planning clinics, school health services, multiservice centers, adolescent clinics, STD clinics, and private practitioners interact daily with adolescents who have already defined a health problem that concerns them. This concern provides an opening for a discussion about AIDS prevention.

How can health providers help young people protect themselves against HIV infection? Some common activities include—

- one-to-one counseling on safer sex, abstinence, or drug use;
- showing films or leading group discussions in waiting rooms;
- distributing appropriate literature on STDs, AIDS, and drugs;
- placing AIDS posters on walls;
- distributing condoms to sexually active clients or those planning to have sex;
- referring patients to telephone hotlines or education programs or other health, mental health, or social services;
- making peer educators available to provide information and referrals.

The goal of these activities is to ensure that every young person who enters the institution will receive multiple messages on AIDS prevention and that the agency defines itself as a place concerned about protecting young people.

Health care institutions can also play an important role in reaching young people at highest risk of HIV infection: runaways and homeless youth, gay youth, young people using IV drugs, and sexually active young people living in neighborhoods with a high prevalence of HIV infection.

These young people often come into contact with agencies such as runaway shelters, youth detention centers, and other social service agencies that provide some health care. Practitioners at these sites must be prepared to raise the issue of AIDS prevention in whatever ways are possible. They also have a special responsibility to become advocates for effective prevention programs in their agencies. The program at Covenant House described earlier in this section illustrates one such program.

Stopping the spread of HIV infection in the next decade depends on AIDS educators' success in reaching young people now. By helping to ensure that every young person has the facts and skills needed to protect himself or herself, AIDS educators can help to spare the generation now coming of age from the ravages of AIDS.

CHAPTER NINE

Women

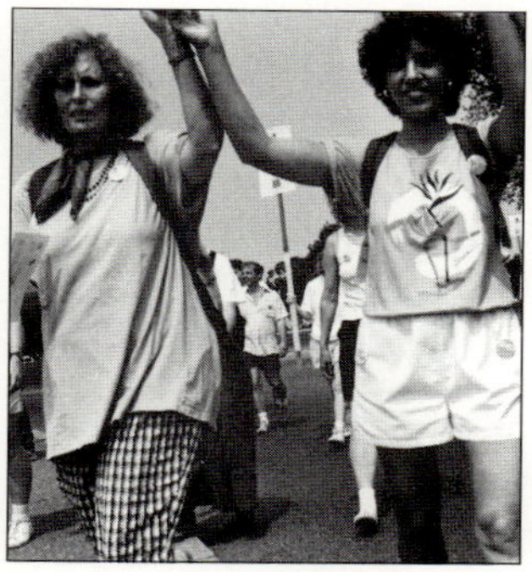

CASE HISTORY

Women's Action Alliance AIDS Project, New York and New Jersey

Founded in 1971, the Women's Action Alliance works to promote equality for women. As a national organization, it helps women and women's organizations around the country by providing information on women's issues, building networks among women's groups, assisting groups in finding the resources needed to strengthen their organizations, and developing new programs on topics not sufficiently addressed by other organizations.

In recent years, the Women's Action Alliance has begun a variety of health projects on issues such as teenage pregnancy prevention and chemical dependency. In November 1987, it began the Women's Center and AIDS Project, designed to help more than 350 community and campus-based multiservice women's centers in New York and New Jersey to develop or improve AIDS programs and services for women. These two states were chosen because of their high proportion of women with AIDS.

Women's centers were chosen as the locations for the program because they service Black, Latina, low-income, and low-opportunity women. Women come to the centers to get job training, parenting support, and services for battered women and to join a variety of support groups. Unlike some other social service agencies, women's centers offer more than categorical programs, thus enabling them to respond to the multiple crises that bring women to their door.

In its first year, the AIDS Project offered several day-long training programs for staff of women's centers in New York and New Jersey. These sessions were designed both to raise the participants' awareness about the impact of AIDS on women and their communities and also to provide a forum for networking and planning action at the local level. Agencies that sent representatives for training included churches, child care centers, battered women's shelters, colleges, hospitals, rape crisis centers, and drug treatment programs. Women who attended reported that the sessions were particularly useful in helping them to understand AIDS as a women's issue.

In its second year, the AIDS Project produced an information packet on AIDS for women's centers. Included in the packet are resource lists of materials and services, education materials appropriate for women, and a desktop guide to relevant organizations and services in each state. In addition to discussing the various ways in which the AIDS epidemic affects women, the guide also describes how to plan AIDS activities such as support groups, outreach programs, and education forums. The packets reinforce and expand the information and skills presented in the training sessions.

In coming years, the Women's Action Alliance AIDS Project plans to provide additional training in New York and New Jersey and to expand to Pennsylvania and Connecticut. It will also provide ongoing technical assistance to the centers that are implementing AIDS programs. Finally, the project will bring together women from centers in different regions to assess the lessons learned from their experience and to plan future directions for their work.

The Scope of the Problem

By the end of 1988, a total of 7,554 adult women had been diagnosed with AIDS in the United States, 9% of the total adult cases. Although the proportion of females with AIDS has remained low from the inception of the epidemic, infected women have attracted special attention. They have been viewed as the major source of infants with AIDS, a group that receives great public sympathy. Women with HIV infection are also seen as an important route for the heterosexual transmission of AIDS—a population group that can facilitate the spread of AIDS beyond the groups where it had previously been concentrated (i.e., gay men and IV drug users).

As is shown later in this chapter, these rationales for concern are epidemiologically problematic, and they can make it more difficult for AIDS educators to involve women in preventive campaigns. Because these beliefs are widespread, however, they constitute an important aspect of the social environment in which AIDS education for women is carried out.

Women with AIDS and HIV Infection

Who are the women with AIDS? More than half are IV drug users and another 30% are sexual partners of a man at risk of AIDS, primarily IV drug users (67%) and bisexual men (16%). Four percent of women with AIDS are sexual partners of men born in countries where AIDS is believed to be transmitted heterosexually, and 11% have contracted AIDS from a blood transfusion. Although the Centers for Disease Control (CDC) does not keep statistics on lesbians with AIDS or HIV infection, the documentation of several cases among lesbians who are not IV drugs users suggests that sexual transmission between women is possible. For women, IV drug use is clearly the single greatest cause of HIV infection.

Women with AIDS tend to be somewhat younger than men with AIDS. It is not surprising that women with AIDS are concentrated in states with serious drug problems: New York, New Jersey, and Florida together account for more than 70% of all female cases of AIDS. In New York City, AIDS is now the leading cause of death for women aged 25 to 34. Nationwide, more than half of women with AIDS are Black and 20% are Latina, a much higher proportion than among men with AIDS.

Serosurveys for HIV antibodies demonstrate varying levels of infection among women. Among IV drug users in New York City, for example, men and women are infected at approximately equal rates, 50% to 60%. For those applying to the military, the ratio of infected men to women was 2.69 to 1; in areas with high infection rates, however, the ratio dropped to 1.21 to 1. Both ratios are considerably lower than the nearly 12-to-1 male-to-female ratio for diagnosed cases of AIDS.

Surveys among female prostitutes show HIV infection rates ranging from zero in Las Vegas to 57% in northern New Jersey. Drug use seems to be the single most important predictor of infection among prostitutes, leading Dr. Molly Coye, health commissioner for the state of New Jersey, to observe that "the surest way to prevent the spread of AIDS through prostitution is to eliminate heroin addiction." More recent evidence suggests that even prostitutes who do not use drugs may be at higher risk if they work in areas of high prevalence of HIV infection.

Surveys for HIV infection among women living in low-income Black and Latino communities in New York City show rates of infectivity of 1% to 5%. Many of these women may not know they are at risk of HIV infection. For example, one study in a municipal hospital in New York City found that 42% of seropositive women who delivered babies had no identifiable risk factor.

Altogether, it is estimated that 100,000 US women are infected with HIV. Some predict that the proportion of women with AIDS will increase significantly. According to the CDC, by 1991 between 8% and 12% of people with AIDS are expected to be women. Whatever the rate of increase, the number of women with AIDS will increase dramatically in the years to come.

Risk Behaviors for Women

To develop effective preventive campaigns, AIDS educators need to understand the specific behaviors and social environments that put women at risk of HIV infection. As the data demonstrate, IV drug use constitutes the greatest threat. The National Institute for Drug Abuse estimates that 350,000 to 400,000 people regularly inject heroin intravenously and perhaps another 1 million inject it occasionally. Of these, slightly more than 500,000 are women.

Female users face even more serious obstacles in getting drug treatment than males. Few programs have special services for women, and almost none provide the child care that many women need if they are to enter treatment. And most programs refuse to treat pregnant women.

Although most female users who are in a hetereosexual relationship have a male partner who is also a drug user, nearly 80% of male drug users are estimated to be in relationships with women who do *not* use drugs. Sexual intercourse with users puts these women at risk of HIV infection, making them an important population for education, especially since many are unaware that their partners are users. Lesbians in relationships with female users are also in need of such education.

Women whose male sex partners are bisexual are also at risk of HIV infection. Data are scarce, but sex researchers estimate that 20% of gay men, or 4 million men, marry at least once. More may have sex with women occasionally. Like the partners of male drug users, women involved with bisexuals are often unaware of their risk. Similarly, some proportion of lesbians have occasional sex with men, including bisexual men, but are often unaware that they are at risk.

Women who have more than one male sex partner, whose partners do not use condoms, and who do not receive regular gynecologic medical care are at higher risk of a number of STDs, including HIV infection. According to a 1982 survey of US women of childbearing age conducted by the National Center for Health Statistics, one out of five women engages in sexual or contraceptive behavior that does not protect her against STDs. Younger women, particularly teenagers, and Black women are less likely to be protected than older women and white women.

Where a woman lives can also affect her risk. In certain Black and Latino neighborhoods in New York City, for example, up to 20% of men are estimated to be infected with HIV. Because most women choose sex partners from their own community, the risk of sexual transmission of HIV in such a neighborhood is much higher than in a low-prevalence area, leading one researcher to observe that "geography is destiny."

Research on gay men suggests that those who engage in sex while under the influence of alcohol or drugs are less likely to practice safer sex. It seems likely that heterosexual women who combine sex and drugs are also at risk, especially women not in stable relationships. Younger women who trade sex for drugs, particularly cocaine, are also unlikely to take action to protect themselves against HIV infection. For this reason, teenage women using crack are believed to be at high risk of HIV infection.

Special Concerns for AIDS Education for Women

Like other groups in need of AIDS education, women are not homogeneous. They have differing values, socioeconomic status, education levels, sexual orientations, and lifestyles. No single intervention can reach all women. Moreover, women fall into many of the other categories described in this section—IV drug user, Black or Latina, youth, disabled—and often this other category provides a more important self-identifier or a better entry point for AIDS education. Nevertheless, some issues in AIDS education are unique for women, and these are considered here.

First, it is women who bear children. Maternal transmission of HIV infection has made women the target of public health planners seeking to slow the rise of pediatric AIDS. Researchers estimate that 30% to 50% of the babies born to infected women will themselves be infected. Although nearly a third of HIV-positive women were infected by a male partner, interventions have focused almost exclusively on the woman herself.

The reason for this focus is the particular social role that women play in reproduction. In our society, women are usually responsible for family planning and contraception. Women also usually carry a disproportionate burden of child care responsibilities. Observing these realities, some AIDS educators suggest that educational interventions must acknowledge these differences. For example, New York City Health Commissioner Stephen Joseph said, "I think women generally have a more sharply defined sense of the future than men. And I think they tend to be more responsible about health issues. This is where we stand a chance of having some success" in AIDS education. With this perspective in mind, many condom promotion campaigns have been targeted at women.

But some disagree with this approach. They believe it reinforces a double standard in which men are encouraged to enjoy their sexuality while women are forced to take responsibility for pregnancy and STDs. The refusal of many organizations, from AIDS groups to the Catholic Church to family planning clinics, to emphasize the contraceptive role as well as the STD-preventing role of condoms imposes an additional burden on women by making them seek two methods of protection rather than relying on condoms (with spermicide) alone.

As noted in the previous section on people of color, African-American and Latina women have their own concerns about reproduction and AIDS. Currently, the CDC recommends that HIV-infected women postpone childbearing indefinitely, a message that for some echoes past calls for forced sterilization and the Tuskegee syphilis experiment (in which Blacks infected with syphilis were denied treatment so that researchers could study the effects of the disease). Suki Ports of New York's Minority Task Force on AIDS noted that urging all women of color to use condoms "can sound genocidal or at least insensitive." Dr. Peter Selwyn, an AIDS doctor at Montefiore Medical Center, observed: "There are people out there who would find it suitable if these women [Blacks and Latinas] stopped having babies altogether. It's too easy to feed into those racist agendas."

Another factor influencing AIDS education in women is their lower social status. Whether one measures it in terms of income, occupational prestige, or numbers of violent attacks, women in this society do less well than men. This status differential has profound implications for AIDS education.

Lack of power can make it difficult for women to persuade their partners to use a condom, stop shooting drugs, or give up other sexual partners. Many women are dependent on men for income and child support. Obviously not all women are in unequal relationships, but sexism is such a pervasive reality that it shapes the values, beliefs, and behaviors of the great majority of men and women.

For many women, AIDS presents a seemingly insoluble dilemma. On the one hand, they are responsible for health protection, contraception, and child care. On the other, they can act in these arenas only in ways that do not violate their partner's pride, masculine self-image, and sense of propriety. Faced with this conundrum, is it surprising that some women respond to the AIDS epidemic with passivity or denial?

Too often, AIDS educators ignore the situation in which women live, reinforcing rather than challenging stereotypes. As Dr. Josette Mondanaro, a Santa Cruz physician who works with female IV drug users, put it, "It would be easy for such women to get the idea from AIDS prevention programs that they are being seen as unclean and, thus, potential spreaders of AIDS to more worthy members of society."

Dr. Constance Wofsy, a physician at San Francisco General Hospital, noted, "To date, women have received more attention for their potential role as infectors than for the problems they face as infectees. Headlines such as 'Nursing Mother Gives Baby AIDS' or 'Infected Hooker Spreads AIDS' contribute to the public perception of women as infectors."

When women, particularly Blacks, Latinas, drug users, or prostitutes, perceive that the goal of AIDS education is to protect society and future generations from them, it is unlikely that such campaigns will get their attention or support.

Recommendations

AIDS educators working with women have developed the following recommendations for reaching this population.

Emphasize that women need to take actions to protect *themselves* from AIDS, not just their partners or their babies.

Not only does such an emphasis provide an additional motivation for preventive action, it also demonstrates that the educators care about the woman as a person, not simply as a transmission vehicle or a vessel for reproduction. The perception of caring is an important prerequisite for credibility and trust. If a woman trusts an educator or a program, she can return for more information, for help in solving problems related to prevention, or for referrals for other services.

Help women use their concerns about AIDS to gain greater control over their lives.

Women's perceptions that they cannot control the circumstances of their life form a primary deterrent to risk-reduction behavior. These are some of the methods that have been used to empower women to win more control:

- Support groups for women at high risk such as IV drug users or partners of bisexuals. Using the consciousness-raising techniques of the early women's movement, these groups provide social support, a sense of solidarity, and a breakdown of isolation. Participants can share successful strategies for practicing safer sex, getting into drug treatment, or ending an unsatisfactory relationship. As one woman who participated in a support group for women affected by AIDS put it, "It helped me to realize I'm somebody."
- Use of peer educators or natural helpers. Female IV drug users, prisoners, prostitutes, and college students have been trained to provide women in similar circumstances with information and skills on AIDS prevention. Use of peers not only increases the credibility of the educator, it also provides learners with a role model.
- Role playing. At a shelter for runaway youth in New York City, young women practice how to convince sexual partners to use a condom. Role plays give participants the opportunity to voice their feelings about their relationships and to develop skills and confidence in negotiating with a partner.

Empowering women helps them use new information on AIDS to protect themselves. It gives them decision-making and negotiating skills that they can use in other settings, and it equips them to play a more active role in educating others about AIDS.

Obviously, no AIDS prevention program can by itself change the status of women. Empowerment programs may not be able to reach women who continue to engage in prostitution to support themselves, to postpone drug treatment because no facility is available, or to stay in an abusive relationship because other options are not viable. In these cases, prevention programs must be able to provide ongoing support to help women survive and protect themselves against AIDS.

Integrate AIDS prevention into existing women's health services.

Family planning and outpatient obstetrics and gynecology clinics, private doctors' offices, and prenatal services provide an ideal opportunity to reach large numbers of women with AIDS prevention messages. Women use these facilities because they are concerned about sexual and reproductive health; they often have an ongoing relationship with a particular provider and are used to discussing at least some aspects of sexual behavior.

Some AIDS prevention activities that women's health services can carry out include—

- distributing pamphlets on AIDS and AIDS prevention;
- showing AIDS films and having a question-and-answer session in the waiting room;
- providing training for staff so that they can offer individual counseling and education on AIDS to their patients;
- displaying posters on AIDS;
- making referrals to AIDS hotlines, support groups, or other relevant services;
- organizing discussion groups for women with concerns about HIV infection;
- offering information, counseling, or referrals on the HIV antibody test;
- distributing condoms and demonstrating their proper use.

Not every site will be able to carry out all these activities, but every women's health service can find some way to educate its patients about AIDS. It is important that these educational approaches also address the specific needs of lesbians for AIDS prevention information.

Use existing channels of communication that reach women to carry AIDS prevention messages.

Effective educators identify the specific media that reach their target population. Among the media that reach various sectors of women are workplace and women's club newsletters; photo novellas; soap operas; women's magazines; lesbian and gay newspapers; parish bulletins; school and college newspapers; talk shows on radio and television; bulletin boards in laundromats, beauty parlors, and supermarkets; and flyers mailed with welfare checks. Each of these has been used to convey information on AIDS.

Because some women at risk of AIDS are hard to reach individually and in geographic communities (e.g., sex partners of male and female IV drug users or bisexuals, and prostitutes), the mass media are important education tools.

Women at risk of HIV infection who are pregnant or considering pregnancy should be provided with nondirective counseling about their options.

The plight of babies with AIDS has led some practitioners and policymakers to believe that they have a moral responsibility to discourage HIV-infected women from reproducing. They argue that the consequences of pediatric AIDS are so devastating and the risk of infection so high that no infected woman should conceive or carry a baby to term.

But others emphasize the importance of allowing women to decide for themselves. Dr. Wendy Chavkin, former director of maternity services and family planning for the New York City Department of Health, described a reproductive choice model for AIDS counseling in which a woman is fully informed about (a) the prognostic implications for herself and for the baby of positive HIV serostatus as well as the associated limitations and uncertainty, (b) the range of possible consequences of positive serostatus for her psychological health and social well-being, and (c) both the burden of the disease and the social support available. Finally, this model requires that whatever choice she makes about the pregnancy be honored and supported.

Dr. Barbara Herbert, a physician and AIDS activist in Baltimore, emphasized this last point. "Unless we can say to women—and mean it—that whatever you choose we will support you concretely, we are not providing them with a choice."

The arguments for nondirective counseling are both ethical and practical. Our legal system emphasizes that the principles of individual privacy and bodily autonomy are violated by any policy of forced pregnancy terminations or sterilization. On more pragmatic grounds, coercion usually drives people away from the health care system, leaving infected women without medical care and with fewer opportunities to learn how to protect themselves and others.

How can health workers dedicated to preventing illness reconcile themselves to supporting an infected woman who chooses to have a baby? Graziela Penchshazadeh, a genetics counselor at New York State Psychiatric Institute, provided a possible answer. "The overall impact of giving people accurate information on perinatal transmission of AIDS, I believe, will be to reduce the number of infected babies born. But in any individual case, my allegiance has to be to the woman I counsel, to help her make the best choice for herself."

Understanding of cultural and religious values can also help the counselor to appreciate that not all women approach the question of whether to risk an infected baby equally. For some women, the ability to have a baby defines their identity as women. Take away that option and self-identity is shattered. Or what of the Pentacostal woman who believes that even five minutes of life will guarantee a baby an eternity in Heaven? Or the Catholic who believes an abortion is a mortal sin?

By accepting that women must make these decisions for themselves, counselors can let go of their personal biases and help their clients make the best decision they can. Services that provide nondirective and supportive counseling will also find that in the long run women will turn to them for help, increasing their ability to provide credible, accurate information. Lesbians who are considering artificial insemination are also in need of education and counseling.

Condom campaigns and safer-sex education should not reinforce a double standard of sexual conduct for men and women.

A sexual ethic that allows men to engage in sex without considering the consequences and requires women to take major responsibility for contraception and disease prevention contributes to the spread of HIV infection. It hinders women from openly discussing risk factors and protective actions with their partners, and it accepts that men cannot be expected to control their sexual impulses. Thus, AIDS educators need to challenge the sexual double standard.

This can be done without resorting to a heavy-handed or moralistic tone. These are some concrete steps that can address this issue:

- Targeting condom campaigns at both men and women.
- Including information on both the contraceptive and STD preventive action of

condoms in all marketing (both these functions are enhanced by combining condoms with a spermicide, such as Nonoxynol-9).

- Teaching skills in communicating about sex to men and women.
- Planning reproductive health services that are attractive and accessible to both men and women.
- Communicating that abstinence and monogamy are viable choices for some men and women. In their appropriate rejection of conservative calls for presenting these two options as the *only* choices, some AIDS educators imply that no healthy adult could choose these paths.

By developing sex education programs that address men's concerns about sexuality, AIDS educators can create a forum to discuss sexual choice. Such an approach will benefit women as well as men.

AIDS education programs for women must respect differences in culture and values on sexuality and gender roles.

One of the dilemmas facing AIDS educators is how to respect the culture and values of diverse populations without reinforcing attitudes or beliefs that contribute to the spread of HIV infection. Machismo, for example, a dominant element of Latino culture, sees the male as superior to the female and encourages female dependence and the deference of women to men in decision making about sexual behavior. Many other cultures (including that of white Americans) have similar though differently expressed values of male dominance and female submission. This issue is discussed more fully in Chapter 7.

Specific recommendations for AIDS education for women are—

- Emphasize values or roles that are positive with respect to prevention—for example, the strong Black woman, Latino men and women protecting each other, the family as a focus for health and sex education.
- Encourage women to assume leadership in AIDS prevention campaigns.
- Create opportunities for women (and men) to discuss culture, sexuality, and health.
- Invite women's organizations (e.g., neighborhood, church, civic, lesbian, and feminist groups) to participate in AIDS prevention activities.

Integrate AIDS education into all services that reach women and link AIDS education to other issues that affect women.

The rationale for developing such connections is twofold. First, many organizations reach women and can play an important role in AIDS prevention. By enabling, for example, school PTAs, drug treatment programs, prisons, churches, and organizations representing prostitutes to take on AIDS prevention, educators magnify their impact on women.

Second, for women to take effective action to prevent HIV infection, they need help in a variety of arenas. Teaching mothers how to talk to their children about AIDS, helping battered women to improve or leave an abusive relationship, or getting an addicted woman into treatment are all measures that can prevent AIDS. Figure 30 lists various organizations that reach women and describes roles they can play in AIDS prevention.

Figure 30. ORGANIZATIONS THAT CAN REACH WOMEN, AND THEIR POTENTIAL ROLES IN AIDS PREVENTION

Organization	Potential Role in Prevention
High schools	Courses on health and sex education; peer education programs.
Colleges	Courses on health and sex education; peer education programs; support groups; condom distribution.
Churches and synagogues	Community forums; women's groups on AIDS; articles in newsletters; projects for social action committees.
Feminist groups	Advocacy for prevention policies that address women's needs; support groups.
Women's civic organizations (e.g., League of Women Voters, Coalition of 100 Black Women)	Community education; education of political leaders; fundraising.
Women's business and professional groups	Education of political leaders; public education; fundraising.
Unions in workplaces with high proportions of women	Workplace education programs; articles in union newspapers.
Family planning clinics and health centers	Counseling, referrals, support groups, medical care, condom distribution and demonstration.
Self-help groups for prostitutes	Advocacy for policies that protect prostitutes; education; support groups.
Drug treatment programs	Advocacy for services that meet special needs of female drug users; education; support groups.
Lesbian organizations	Education of lesbians; advocacy for programs to meet their needs.
Child care centers	Education of parents.
Employment training programs	Education and referrals.
AIDS organizations	Community education aimed at women; training and technical assistance to women's groups.

C H A P T E R   T E N

Workers

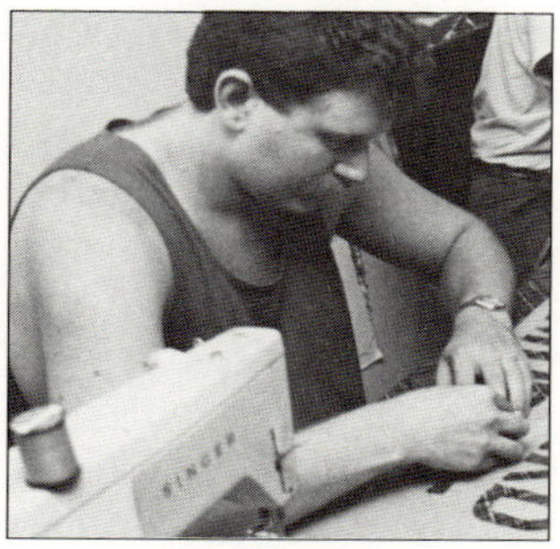

CASE HISTORY

Levi Strauss, San Francisco

In 1982, a few employees of Levi Strauss, the jeans manufacturer with corporate headquarters in San Francisco, asked Robert D. Haas, the chief executive, for permission to distribute AIDS information in the lobby of the main office. In an unusual move that presaged the company's pioneering role in AIDS education, Haas and other senior management helped staff the information table, demonstrating their own and the company's concern about AIDS. "As employers," observed Haas, "we have the responsibility to maintain an open and informed working environment that at least combats unwarranted employee fears and prejudices."

To achieve this end, Levi Strauss has developed a comprehensive education program that includes—

- *training for managers and staff personnel on AIDS issues and related company policy;*
- *establishment of an interdepartmental AIDS task force that advises the company on AIDS issues;*
- *production of a videotape on AIDS for staff and other employers;*
- *lunchtime lectures on AIDS open to all employees;*

- articles on AIDS and prevention in its health and fitness newsletter;
- conferences on workplace AIDS education for other companies.

Levi Strauss has not limited its activities to education. To create an institutional climate that supports a compassionate and effective response to the AIDS epidemic, the company has instituted several policies that protect its employees:

- The corporation bans discrimination against HIV-infected employees. Those with AIDS have the same benefits, medical coverage, and right to work as anyone else with a serious illness.
- Employees with AIDS can stay on the job as long as possible, with some options for part-time or flexible work schedules.
- Home health care is available for employees who need it.
- Strict guidelines protect the confidentiality of employees with AIDS.
- A corporate foundation donates money to AIDS-related organizations.

Levi Strauss's program has been very successful in its San Francisco office, but resistance in other facilities, particularly in the South, has been strong. "We've had some struggles out in the field," noted Robert Dunn, vice-president for corporate communications and community affairs.

To address this problem, the company's AIDS educators have looked for new ways to raise the issue. "In the South," said Roberta Rich-Johnson, a medical specialist with the Levi Strauss Employee Assistance Program, "there's a lot of teenage pregnancy, so clearly those kids are having unprotected sex. We're trying to get through the AIDS issue by using teenage sexuality. We're talking to parents about how to talk to your kids about sexuality."

Dr. Alan Emery, a psychologist with the San Francisco AIDS Foundation, has called Levi Strauss "the pioneer in creating a responsible, ethical and humane AIDS program." Whether other corporations will be able to emulate its commitment remains to be seen.

CASE HISTORY

AIDS Education at the Service Employees International Union

The Service Employees International Union (SEIU) represents 850,000 workers; more than a third of its members are health care workers. Since 1983, SEIU has been in the forefront of unions addressing the AIDS issue. In that year, Local 250, representing 30,000 health care workers in northern California, organized its rank-and-file AIDS education committee.

In the past five years, Local 250 has sponsored a variety of activities:

- Committee members helped plan and conduct union-sponsored AIDS education workshops for staff, stewards, and interested members.
- Committee members have served on the AIDS task forces of several hospitals, helping to review hospitals' AIDS policies and protocols.
- Members of the AIDS committee have become advocates for AIDS patients, helping to find resources and staff for designated AIDS units at certain hospitals.

Figure 32. POLICY QUESTIONS ON AIDS FOR EMPLOYERS

- Should employees be tested for HIV infection?
- Should new employees be tested?
- Should people with AIDS be fired?
- Should employees who refuse to serve people with AIDS be disciplined?
- Should employees have the right to refuse working with people with AIDS?
- Should employees who refuse to work with or near people with AIDS be disciplined?
- How can the employer fulfill legal responsibilities to protect employees from HIV infection?
- What legal obligation do employers have to provide AIDS education?
- What responsibilities do employers have to protect the confidentiality of their employees' medical status?

of the policy issues that employers must consider before implementing education programs.

Common Questions Faced by Workplace AIDS Educators

This section poses some of the questions that workplace AIDS educators have faced and provides the answers their experience has suggested.

Who should sponsor workplace AIDS education programs?

Workplace AIDS programs have been sponsored by management, by unions, by outside organizations, and by combinations of the three. The case histories illustrate two of these approaches. Each has its unique advantages and disadvantages.

Management-run programs have clear authority to provide education to all levels of workers. Corporate support also helps to ensure that necessary resources are available. As Roberta Rich-Johnson, a medical specialist in the Employee Assistance Program at Levi Strauss, explained, "This company sees itself as having a corporate responsibility. It is management's position to do something about AIDS because it has to come from above; it has to be important enough for management to make a commitment to it, because otherwise AIDS education won't work."

Companies that already have an employee assistance program, a medical office, or some health education services can use this existing structure to provide AIDS education and thereby reduce the need to create new organizational forms. Moreover, existing channels of communication often have a familiarity and acceptability that special AIDS materials lack. The CBS Corporation, for example, devoted an issue of its wellness programs newsletter to AIDS prevention, thereby providing accurate information to thousands of employees. And because companies have a strong financial incentive to maintain their employees' health, their commitment to AIDS prevention may be high.

On the other hand, management-run programs may lack credibility with workers, another example of the preexisting tensions that so often influence AIDS education. "Our experience has been that employers use education as another tool to get their employees to do what they're supposed to do," said a health and safety staff person for a major national union. "As a result, many workers are not likely to listen when the company assures them that there are no risks in the workplace but they better watch out who they have sex with and how and they better stop using drugs." The very fact that management has a financial stake in keeping its workers healthy or in excluding sick employees may make workers feel the company's motives are economic rather than medical.

In companies where management denies that AIDS is a real or potential problem, management may be unwilling to make the commitment to develop an effective program. A 1985 survey by the American Management Association found that only 15% of the 124 companies questioned were attempting to educate their employees. Only 4% had created any formal AIDS policies.

AIDS education programs run by labor unions may address some of the problems of credibility and commitment. As Alan Lubin of New York City's United Federation of Teachers explained: "Teachers will accept information about AIDS from the union quicker than they will accept it from the Board of Education. That's management coming in to say, 'Don't worry, you might die, but we'll protect you,' and there's a lack of trust. There's no lack of trust with the UFT, and they'll accept messages from us."

As the description of the SEIU AIDS program demonstrated, large national unions have the resources to develop education materials, provide technical assistance to local chapters, and advocate policies that support prevention. Unions that represent workers caring for people with AIDS have already developed a variety of AIDS education programs.

However, fewer than 20% of workers in the United States belong to unions, and some unions lack either the resources or the commitment to address AIDS issues. For workers in these settings, union-sponsored programs are not a realistic option.

Many workplace AIDS educators believe that joint worker-management education programs offer the best hope for effective interventions. Elaine Askari of the Labor Occupational Health Program at the University of California at Berkeley explained, "AIDS is something that unions and management can work together on in a non-adversarial way." The advantages of this approach are that all affected parties are involved in planning, implementing, and evaluating programs; that the committee becomes a forum for raising policy-related AIDS issues; and that emerging problems can be identified early and corrected.

Regardless of who sponsors a program, management support is essential. Workers need release time to attend training, and mid-level supervisors need to reinforce messages conveyed in programs. For those workers who provide services to HIV-infected people that could result in exposure to body fluids, management is responsible for providing gloves and other protective equipment. All these issues can be discussed by joint management-worker committees.

Still another option for workplace AIDS education is to invite an outside agency to provide training. The American Red Cross, for example, will send speakers, videos, and materials to employers who request them. Often health departments and voluntary AIDS organizations offer these services, too. By inviting appropriate outside experts, workplace programs can increase the credibility of education and diminish the perception of conflict of interest that sometimes greets in-house programs. A potential problem of packaged AIDS education programs is that they may not address the specific concerns of employees in a particular setting. Previewing such programs and adding additional components (e.g., guest speakers) can address these concerns.

How can AIDS educators convince an employer or union to begin a program?

"Some companies are afraid that if you talk about AIDS, people are going to get afraid, as if they're not already afraid," reported Judy Spiegel of AIDS Project Los Angeles. "It's like parents not wanting to talk to their kids about sex for fear that it'll make them start doing it."

As in every other setting, fear and denial are major obstacles blocking workplace AIDS programs. Unfortunately, it is often a crisis—an employee who is discovered to have AIDS or a worker refusing to care for a person with AIDS—that first leads to action. New England Telephone and Telegraph Company, for example, began an AIDS education program only after an employee with AIDS reached an out-of-court settlement in a lawsuit charging discrimination and breach of privacy.

By alerting employers to the financial, social, and legal costs of *not* implementing a program, educators can sometimes persuade them to take action. Another strategy is to provide information about existing corporate programs. Learning that many Fortune 500 companies have already provided their employees with AIDS education may convince a chief executive that such programs are not radical. For smaller companies, the availability of packaged programs from credible organizations like the American Red Cross may lower the financial and social costs of implementing AIDS education.

Similarly, the availability of model union-based programs, combined with increasing demands for information from union members, may convince labor unions to establish AIDS education programs.

How can workplace programs diminish fear and hysteria?

AIDS educators with workplace experience suggest several steps that can maximize the impact of such programs.

First, AIDS education programs should begin *before* a crisis arises. Participants are more receptive, personal fears are lower, and workers and management are less likely to have staked out inflexible positions.

Second, all levels of workers should receive training. In health care institutions, for example, not only nurses and doctors but also housekeeping, food service, and laundry staff require AIDS education. "We found out that unless we included telephone receptionists in our program," reported one AIDS educator training a health center staff in Philadelphia, "the patients' first encounter with the system might undermine our whole effort." Similarly, management needs to be trained in order to support the goals of the education program. The uninformed or prejudiced remarks of one supervisor can set an example that undercuts weeks of education.

Third, all levels of participants need to have input into the content and form of the educational intervention. What works for professional employees may not work for nonprofessionals. Only by talking to workers before the training begins can educators assess what learners know and what they need to know. Further, by consulting participants before education, educators give learners a stake in the program. This is particularly important in settings where workers may distrust a management-sponsored program.

Fourth, AIDS education must be a part of (not a substitute for) a more comprehensive approach to AIDS in the workplace. Management's responsibility to provide workers with protective equipment (e.g., gloves or masks), protocols for infection control, and a clear policy on the rights of workers with AIDS are among the issues that must be addressed. In the absence of clear written guidelines, education can become a source of frustration rather than improvement.

Finally, AIDS education programs need an ongoing presence in the workplace. One lecture or one pamphlet is not sufficient. In Bellevue Hospital in New York City, the hospital with more AIDS patients than any other in the United States, the AIDS educator gave a 45-minute lecture to all new employees. But she also gave out her telephone number so that workers with a question could reach her (or an answering machine) to get additional information when they needed it. Her ready accessibility, she believed, helped to prevent many problems that unanswered questions might create.

Should workplace programs separate employees by job title, or are institution-wide programs more effective?

"If I'm a food service worker and you're a food service worker, I'm more likely to believe what you tell me than a doctor or someone from management," reported Elaine Askari. Based on an evaluation of an AIDS education program for health care workers of various kinds in Boston, program planners recommended "special educational programs directed at each group, taking into account preexisting differences in knowledge and attitudes." But an AIDS educator working for a union in New York City said, "We have found that by including all job titles and management in our AIDS education sessions, we have created a forum for discussing the issues that come up in the workplace. By separating groups, we would have lost that opportunity."

These quotes illustrate the range of opinions on targeted versus generic workplace programs. Perhaps the two are not mutually exclusive approaches: Systemic issues such as discrimination, fear, and the establishment of protocols can best be addressed in groups that include all types of workers. Specific information on the risks and protective actions required in particular job settings can be better addressed by bringing together all these in one job title. Developing a cadre of educators with backgrounds in relevant job settings, as SEIU did in Northern California, can help ensure that education is appropriate.

Among the issues educators need to consider in deciding which approach to use are the credibility of the communicator, the extent to which the educator understands the day-to-day realities of various job titles, the impact of other participants on the learning process, and cost factors.

Should AIDS education programs be voluntary or mandatory?

Forcing people to attend education programs against their will diminishes the likelihood of effective learning. On the other hand, failing to provide employees with information or skills they need to protect themselves or to deliver mandated services may constitute employer negligence.

Mandatory programs require all workers to be exposed to AIDS prevention messages. According to Judy Spiegel of AIDS Project Los Angeles, "Employees are afraid that if they show up at an optional AIDS training session, or (God forbid) ask a question, people will begin to wonder about them. That's why it is important that the sessions be mandatory."

It may be possible to distinguish among program objectives: Some activities should be mandatory whereas others can be voluntary. For example, information on infection control measures, discrimination, and delegation of the responsibilities of workers and management should probably be provided to all workers. Personal examination of one's feelings and attitudes, and development of private risk-reduction strategies may have to be voluntary. By providing access to employee assistance programs or an outside organization, employers can ensure that all who want more information or counseling can get it.

When AIDS education programs are mandatory, it is essential that employers make them as accessible as possible. Attendance should be during paid company time (not during lunch hours or breaks), and the quality of the programs should be high. Mandatory attendance at boring, superficial, or insensitive programs can create resentment and resistance.

What methods of workplace education are effective?

Workplace AIDS education programs have used the range of strategies described in earlier chapters: films and videos, pamphlets, lectures, small group discussions, counseling, and so on. But according to Dale Feurer, a contributing editor of *Training* magazine, "The consensus among consultants and in-house practitioners alike is that stand-up training is the best way to approach AIDS education." Roberta Rich-Johnson of Levi Strauss agreed: "In our experience, direct training is essential because people have questions that require immediate answers."

For programs for professionals, educators suggest that the trainer come from the same discipline as the learners. "Health workers learn best from their own kind," explained Dennis James, health care educator for the AIDS Action Committee in Boston, "so we have nurses educate nurses and physicians educate physicians." Elaine Askari of the Labor Occupational Health Program trained nonprofessional health workers to educate their co-workers about AIDS.

What are the special needs of health care workers for AIDS education?

More than any other group, health care workers are likely to have repeated or extended interactions with people with AIDS or HIV infection. A variety of studies show that there is a low but measurable risk of HIV infection for those who are accidentally injected with contaminated blood and for those who have infected blood or other body fluids spilled or splashed on open wounds or on mucous membranes.

According to CDC, by mid-1988, 20 health care workers or people who provide care to infected patients seem to have contracted HIV infection through workplace exposure. Various research teams in the United States and Canada have followed 2,663 health care workers who have had needle-stick injuries or spills or splashes of infected blood. Thus far, five of these people (about 2 per 1,000) have tested positive for HIV infection. Still another study of 270 health care workers at San Francisco General Hospital, 75% of whom had treated AIDS patients at least a year before the study, found that none had seroconverted.

These data have led CDC to recommend that health care workers in contact with body fluids follow recommended infection control measures to further lower their risk. In November 1987, a joint advisory letter of the US Public Health Service and the Department of Labor mandated that health care institutions must follow these guidelines.

Coping with the anxiety that this risk poses is without doubt the most significant issue that AIDS education programs for health care workers must address. AIDS educators have developed several strategies to help workers respond to their fears appropriately.

First, education programs must provide employees with an opportunity to voice their fears. "Many of the people we talk to know the facts already," reported Dennis James, "so we concentrate on emotions. Unless people's fears and phobias are up for discussion, the information we have to impart won't make a difference." Attempting to reassure health workers solely by presenting data with no opportunity to discuss fears is an ineffective strategy.

Second, workers need specific instructions in infection control practices. They need to understand the rationale for protective measures so that they can take appropriate steps to deal with real threats (e.g., internal exposure to body fluids) without refusing to provide needed services, such as delivering a food tray to a person with AIDS. Moreover, management must ensure that all protective equipment is readily available when and where it is needed.

Third, some educators have found that linking AIDS prevention to other infectious disease control measures seems to be effective. Richard Goldberg, an AIDS educator with the Los Angeles County Department of Health, explained: "The techniques we've used, for example, to work with dentists, is *not* to separate AIDS out as a special issue but to show them that it's part and parcel of general concerns of infection control. When you show them they already know all the techniques and procedures they will ever need to deal with a person with AIDS, they seem to say, well, okay. As long as they perceive AIDS as something special and extraordinary, they're not prepared to do the work." Many more health workers contract hepatitis B in the workplace than HIV.

Fourth, health care workers who care for people with AIDS or HIV infection also need ongoing support to help them cope with their fears. Not only is there the specific fear of contracting HIV, there is also the fear of death that caring for young people who are dying often evokes. Added to these emotions are the grief of losing so many patients and the anguish of seeing people suffer. Together these feelings can make health care workers feel overwhelmed, frightened, and depressed.

Some AIDS units have established support groups for their workers where these experiences can be shared and analyzed. Others make individual counseling available. As the caseload of people with AIDS increases, health care institutions will need to make greater efforts to provide the range of support services that AIDS caregivers require.

C H A P T E R   E L E V E N

Prisoners

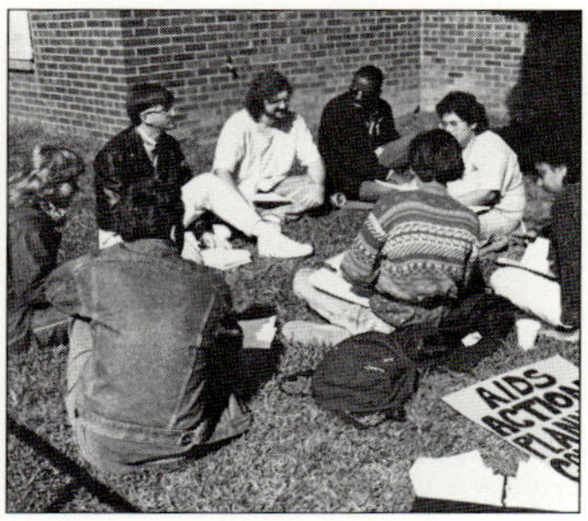

At the end of 1986, 3.2 million people in the United States were behind bars, on probation, or on parole. About 820,000 of these were actually in prison or jail. Because many prisoners are current or former drug users, the correctional system offers excellent opportunities for AIDS prevention. For many young adults, especially African-Americans and Latinos, it is the dominant social institution in their lives. In this way, prisons and jails provide one of the best ways to reach people who are often bypassed by public health programs.

According to a survey of correctional systems conducted by the National Institute of Justice, an arm of the US Department of Justice, 3,136 prisoners had been diagnosed with AIDS as of October 1988. Of these, 59% were in New York, New Jersey, and Pennsylvania, all states with a significant drug problem. Prisoners with AIDS are more likely to be IV drug users and more likely to be Black and Latino than the population with AIDS outside prison. In the New York state prison system, for example, 95% of those with AIDS were IV drug users. It is estimated that 60% of all prisoners in that system have used IV drugs. Although the prevalence of AIDS among prisoners is somewhat higher than in the rest of the population (probably due to high rates of IV drug use), the rate of increase in prisons is lower. The National Institute of Justice report concluded that AIDS is rarely transmitted in prison. Rather, inmates who were infected before incarceration become ill during their stay.

Serosurveys of inmates show wide variation in the prevalence of HIV infection. In federal prisons, where HIV testing is now mandatory, rates in 1988 were 1.7% for released males and 1.3% for released females. Rates for new inmates were somewhat higher. In low-incidence areas, the prevalence of infection is also very low; in Iowa, for example, 0.2% of inmates were found to be positive in 1988. In Los Angeles, about 15% of inmates are seropositive. And it is estimated that nearly a quarter of the 50,000 inmates seen at Rikers Island, the detention facility in New York City, are HIV infected.

Because both sexual activity and drug use are illegal in prison, good data on the prevalence of risk behaviors are unavailable. In a report prepared for the National Institute of Justice, Theodore Hammett estimated that from 9% to 20% of inmates were targets of aggressive sexual acts during their incarceration. Probably more engage in consensual sexual activity. As well as sharing needles for drug use, some prisoners are tattooed during their incarceration by other inmates, often with unsterile needles.

Goals for AIDS Education in Prisons

AIDS educators working in prisons have identified the following goals:

- Provide inmates, guards, and other staff with accurate information on AIDS and its prevention.
- Help prisoners develop AIDS prevention skills that can protect them in prison and after their release.
- Help prison officials develop preventive policies and programs that are humane and effective.
- Reduce unnecessary fears and hysteria about AIDS among inmates, guards, and prison officials.
- Help prevent discrimination against people who have AIDS, who are HIV infected, or who are perceived to be HIV infected.

Obstacles to AIDS Education in Prisons

Dr. Charles Braslow, medical director at Riker's Island Detention Center in New York City, summarized the advantages of the prison setting for AIDS education:

> *Correctional facilities provide a particularly auspicious location for such efforts since they contain a concentration of drug users who are removed from states of drug intoxication and drug-seeking behavior and so are likely to benefit from educational efforts. Equally important, lessons learned inside are not forgotten outside, resulting in an increased level of knowledge "in the streets" after discharge. These "street" drug abusers have so far been a difficult population for AIDS educators to reach, and correctional facilities can be a major focal point in targeting them for risk reduction.*

Prisoners are the prototypical captive population; AIDS education can provide a welcome relief from the boredom of prison routine, and educators can develop a relationship with learners that is not possible in more transient populations.

Despite these advantages, AIDS educators in prisons face formidable obstacles. The authoritarian atmosphere is one obvious impediment. To develop education programs that help learners gain greater control over their lives in a setting designed to emphasize their lack of freedom presents educators with a nearly insoluble dilemma.

Security concerns further restrict educators. They dictate the timing, setting, and participants in any education session. They make it difficult to involve family members or to maintain ongoing contact with prisoners who can be transferred from one site to another, often without notice.

For many prisoners, fear of violence from other inmates or guards dominates their lives, making them inaccessible for education. An inmate who is identified as being HIV infected, or even interested in AIDS, may be subject to physical reprisals from other inmates. As Billy Jones and Eugene Philyaw, AIDS educators with Whitman-Walker Clinic in Washington, DC, noted, "Prisoners coexist in stressful and hostile environments of classism, racism, sexism, and homophobia—environments in which the primary means of coping and expressing emotions are via sex, drugs, and violence."

Prison officials often have negative attitudes toward AIDS education. Like officials in other settings, they can see AIDS prevention as one more burden to be added to a mission that is already impossible. In addition, given a choice between coercive strategies such as mandatory testing and isolation of infected inmates and comprehensive AIDS education, many officials will choose the former. Larry Gostin, executive director of the American Society of Law and Medicine, observed: "While the real challenge is to discover and prevent unhealthy behavior, prison resources are being increasingly used instead to detect who is seropositive and who is not." When prisoners perceive that a program's primary goal is to label and isolate certain individuals, it is unlikely that AIDS educators will be trusted.

In some cases, prisoners have challenged officials' reluctance to provide AIDS education. John Sheridan, a New Jersey inmate and a prisoner rights advocate, sued the state Department of Corrections for what he called its refusal to provide risk-reduction information. Corrections officials "are treating this like it's a criminal justice issue," he said, "and it's not. It's a health issue. If this is important public health information that every citizen should have, then why shouldn't prisoners have it?" Class action lawsuits in Connecticut and Alabama are also seeking to force corrections departments to provide adequate AIDS education.

Prison guards and other inmates often reinforce unrealistic fears about HIV transmission. When inmates see guards wearing gloves and masks for routine handling of infected prisoners, they do not believe reassurances that the virus is difficult to transmit. Jordan Barab, a safety and health coordinator of the American Federation of Federal, State, County, and Municipal Employees (a union representing 50,000 corrections employees), observed: "It's perfectly understandable that people are going to have hysterical reactions not based on fact if they haven't been educated. We're dealing with more than reality; we're dealing with perception here." And as one inmate warned, "There is going to be a riot here and it's going to be because of AIDS."

Finally, public officials sometimes oppose AIDS prevention policies for prisons. Efforts to distribute condoms to inmates or to teach them how to sterilize needles have been blocked by officials who believe such actions condone illegal activities. For example, in response to a plan to distribute condoms to gay prisoners in the city's detention centers, the New York City Council majority leader said, "It's stupid. They broke some laws to be put in jail and now they are being told it's okay to further break laws."

The very factors that make AIDS education in prisons so difficult emphasize its importance. Increasingly, prison officials are realizing the costs of *not* educating staff and inmates about AIDS. This new understanding may create openings for AIDS educators to play a role in developing effective programs.

Recommendations

Include prison officials in the planning of education programs and educate them about the complexity of AIDS.

Getting the support and understanding of prison officials is a critical first step in implementing AIDS education programs. Before Health Education Research Organization (HERO), the Baltimore AIDS organization, began its work in Maryland prisons, its staff met with the management of the state Department of Corrections. As a result of these discussions, reported HERO's Bobby Klihis, "Our relations with the Department of Corrections have been wonderful." However, in other cases, prison officials have strongly resisted efforts to initiate education programs, even when efforts were made to involve them directly.

Billy Jones and Eugene Philyaw of Washington, DC's Whitman-Walker Clinic listed the questions they asked at meetings with prison administrators and medical personnel:

- What education strategies regarding AIDS, sex, drugs, and tattoos are currently implemented?
- Are sexual minorities isolated, housed in protective custody units, or under some other arrangements?
- Are inmates routinely tested for HIV antibodies?
- Have correctional officers received any specific training regarding HIV issues?
- Are people who test positive isolated?
- Are medical, psychological, and social services provided to those who test positive or have ARC or AIDS or both?

Answers to these inquiries suggest the content and goals of subsequent education programs.

Begin education programs with training for corrections officers and staff.

Corrections officers interact with inmates daily and will continue to see them long after the AIDS educators have moved on. Their attitudes and behaviors with respect to HIV infection will profoundly influence the climate in prison.

At the Whitman-Walker Clinic, prison educators insist that before agreeing to conduct seminars for inmates, they must educate corrections officers and other staff. At a minimum, officers must be able to answer inmates' questions accurately. AIDS educators spend four hours with correctional officers. "Anything less," they said, "doesn't permit anxiety issues to be addressed."

Bobby Klihis of HERO noted that "training guards is a hard nut to crack," because many are resistant to any discussion of AIDS. In her experience, guards who are forced to attend training are "not as receptive" as volunteers. The New York State Department of Corrections, on the other hand, has mandated AIDS in-service training for all correctional system personnel, as well as preservice training in their training academy. Depending on the nature of that training, such a policy can help ensure that all staff receive accurate information.

Identify those prison issues that can be addressed by education and those that cannot.

Like officials in other settings, some prison administrators hope that an AIDS education program can solve all their institution's AIDS problems. This a vain hope. Education is certainly a necessary component of an institutional response, but it is hardly sufficient. Among the issues that are *not* likely to be solved by education are the following:

- What services will the prison provide for HIV-infected inmates, and will those inmates be isolated?
- What will the institution's policy be on HIV testing?
- How will the prison discourage sexual attacks and illicit drug use?
- What guidelines will determine how staff respond to infected inmates and those perceived to be infected?
- How will the confidentiality of prisoners' medical status be protected?
- Will the prison provide drug detoxification services for addicted inmates?

Health educators can play an important role in helping institutions to set policy on these issues, but they cannot resolve them on their own. By making clear the limits of their expertise and the potential impact of their interventions, AIDS educators can prevent unrealistic expectations or disappointment with unachieved goals.

Develop testing programs that maximize the educational impact of the test.

AIDS educators will usually not have a decisive voice in shaping screening policies. In the federal system, for example, the order for mandatory testing came directly from the White House.

Many prison health officials question the wisdom of mandatory testing. Dr. Charles Braslow of Rikers Island argued against such a policy because "there is not evidence that rates of transmission are higher in correctional facilities than in the general population"; because confidentiality is difficult to maintain, resulting in potential risk to personal safety in the prison and discrimination outside; and because widespread testing "diverts scarce resources from more effective educational efforts." In the San Francisco County Jail, HIV testing is offered only to pregnant women because the medical administration does not believe informed consent is possible in a correctional facility. In the state of Alabama, however, a law mandating HIV testing for all inmates was enacted in 1987.

But whatever the testing policy, educators should include these essential elements of a screening program:

- pretest counseling about the significance of the test;
- referrals for needed health, mental health, and social services;
- posttest counseling for both positives and negatives;
- risk-reduction education on safer sex and drug use;
- ongoing medical and support services for those who are seropositive;
- measures to ensure confidentiality of results.

Without these elements, it is questionable whether a screening program will meet acceptable ethical standards of public health practice. By ensuring that inmates have the opportunity to benefit personally from testing programs, AIDS educators can contribute to the programs' educational impact.

Develop education programs for all institutions in the correctional system.

Because prisons with long-term inmates have the most stable populations and routines, it is often easier to add AIDS prevention programs there than in short-term detention centers. But facilities holding people before sentencing have larger populations, including many people arrested for drug use or prostitution. They provide an important opportunity to reach those who may never be sentenced and are unlikely to come into contact with other public health programs. For many drug users, it may be their sole contact with an AIDS prevention program.

Similarly, juvenile detention centers, halfway houses, and parole programs can bring prevention messages to new populations or reinforce education offered in other correctional settings. Training staff throughout the correctional system—police officers, judges, guards, parole officers, educators, and health providers—ensures a more uniform response to inmates' concerns and questions. By developing a system-wide plan for correctional institutions, AIDS educators can help guarantee that anyone who sets foot in a prison or jail gets some AIDS education.

To address the thorny bureaucratic and political problems that arise in planning for local, state, and federal institutions, it is often helpful to convene a task force that includes representatives from all appropriate agencies and advocacy groups. Such a task force will not usually have decision-making power, but it can prod administrators to coordinate their response to the AIDS epidemic. It can also encourage frontline educators to share experiences and problems.

Include prisoners in planning and implementing prison AIDS education programs.

An educator who has spent time behind bars may have added credibility. AIDS programs have used a peer approach in several ways. Inmates at a New York State prison produced a film on AIDS called "A Bad Way to Die." It included interviews with prisoners with AIDS and several experts. At the inmates' insistence, the fear message was emphasized. In Baltimore, HERO sponsored a competition for the best AIDS poster created by an inmate. Participation in the contest was high.

HERO in Baltimore, the Association for Drug Abuse Prevention and Treatment (ADAPT) in New York City, and other groups have used ex-inmates to educate prisoners about AIDS. In some correctional facilities, prisoners themselves have educated each other about AIDS, filling an institutional vacuum. Most AIDS education programs are enthusiastic about this approach, arguing that current and ex-inmates sidestep the class, race, and power issues that professionals encounter. But Bobby Klihis of HERO reported that peer educators were not always credible sources of medical information, and so some inmates ignored their message. Any effective program requires careful training of peer educators. Pending more rigorous evaluations of various strategies, a sensible course might be to include both professionals and peer educators in any program.

Integrate AIDS education into prison drug detoxification programs.

Recent research shows that offering drug detoxification and drug treatment to inmates significantly reduces the likelihood of subsequent arrest. Since other studies show that half to three quarters of men arrested for serious crimes in major urban areas have recently used illicit drugs, the potential benefits of improved drug treatment in the correctional system seems high.

Such programs are also a critical focal point for AIDS education. In New York City, for example, all addicted inmates who pass through Rikers Island, the city's detention facility, are referred to the drug detoxification unit. Several full-time AIDS educators run groups, provide counseling, and distribute education materials. By helping prison officials include AIDS education in any new drug treatment programs, educators can reach a population at very high risk of HIV infection.

Address the special needs of female inmates.

Because prisoners are overwhelmingly male, prisons have been slow to meet the special needs of their growing female population. Yet one study in Maryland found that 15% of new female inmates were HIV infected compared to 7% of newly jailed males. The higher rate among women was attributed to their higher prevalence of IV drug use.

Because a very high proportion of arrested females are charged with drug crimes or prostitution, female inmates may be at high risk of HIV infection. Prostitutes who use IV drugs are at higher risk of HIV infection than those who do not.

Among the special AIDS-related needs of female inmates are—

- availability of HIV testing and extensive counseling for pregnant inmates (see Chapter 9, "Women");
- education on safer sex and perinatal transmission of AIDS (men need this, too, but programs for women must address their own specific concerns and the power issues discussed in Chapter 9);
- access to drug detoxification and AIDS treatment programs open to women;
- a discussion of the potential for lesbians who use drugs to infect their partners through sexual transmission.

Develop a comprehensive plan to protect the confidentiality of medical information about prisoners.

Perhaps in no other setting are the consequences of revealing a person's health status more drastic than in prison. Inmates who are identified as HIV infected have been beaten, isolated, shunned, and ostracized. For an inmate who actually has AIDS or ARC, coping with the prison system's response to the diagnosis as well as with the disease and incarceration adds a staggering burden.

AIDS educators usually do not have the power to make rules about confidentiality. But they can educate administrators about the consequences of breaches, and they can make sure their own practice does not endanger their clients.

Some prison AIDS educators report that inmates were reluctant to talk to them for fear of being stigmatized. Mandating AIDS education for all prisoners is one method of overcoming this problem. Placing the educator in the prison health service is another; inmates can then request to see a health provider and be offered AIDS counseling in a more private setting.

Perhaps the most effective strategy for protecting confidentiality is a comprehensive education program for inmates, staff, and administrators that helps to allay fears about transmission and increase understanding of the importance of confidentiality.

CHAPTER TWELVE

People with Hemophilia and Other Blood Disorders

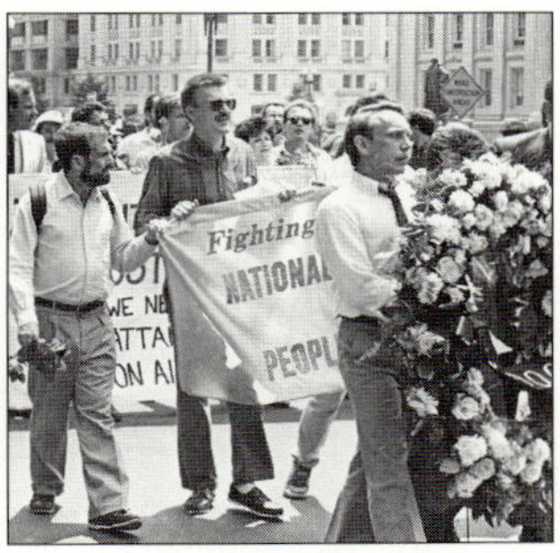

Extent of AIDS Among Hemophiliacs

Between 15,000 and 20,000 Americans have hemophilia, an inherited bleeding disorder. It is estimated that 40% to 70% of these have been infected with HIV by the blood products that they take to save their lives. Researchers estimate that 10% to 20% of the steady sex partners of infected hemophiliacs are also infected. Nearly 800 hemophiliacs and those with other blood disorders had been diagnosed with AIDS by the end of 1988, 1% of the total US cases. Although heat treatments now kill HIV in blood products, minimizing the risk to uninfected hemophiliacs, important goals for AIDS educators are to educate hemophiliacs about HIV infection and support their families and those that interact with them.

For hemophiliacs, like every group affected by AIDS, the disease has become one more burden added to an already heavy load. "The real tragedy," explained Dr. Margaret Hillgartner, the physician who directs the hemophilia clinic at New York Hospital, "is the fact that we had thought these people would lead relatively normal lives with the development of [blood] concentrates. It seems so unfair. The majority have learned to come to grips with hemophilia. They have gone to school, gotten jobs, married, started families. Now that is knocked out from under them." Or as one young man put it, "Hemophilia was something I had all my life, a condition I had continually to adjust to. . . . AIDS is an atom blast overnight."

AIDS educators working with hemophiliacs have suggested the following goals for education programs:

- Provide eduation on transmission of HIV infection.
- Teach safer-sex techniques.
- Emphasize the importance of general health promotion measures such as good nutrition, adequate rest, and avoidance of drugs and alcohol.
- Develop skills in discussing sexual practices with partners.
- Discuss the potential for discrimination and the remedies available to combat it.
- Help learners to develop strategies for discussing their conditions (both hemophilia and HIV status) with others in a way that prevents disease, maximizes social interactions, and reduces discrimination.

All those who come into regular contact with hemophiliacs, such as their families, friends, teachers, classmates, and health care providers, also need education in these areas.

Recommendations

AIDS educators working with hemophiliacs make the following suggestions for effective education for this population.

Integrate AIDS education into comprehensive care of hemophiliacs.

Most hemophiliacs are connected to an ongoing medical care program. This provides a natural forum for AIDS prevention messages. As Christopher Whitney, director of AIDS education for the National Hemophilia Foundation, noted, "People with hemophilia tend to trust doctors and the medical world," making them a credible source of information.

Effective integration of AIDS education requires AIDS training for medical providers working with hemophiliacs. The National Hemophilia Foundation and other organizations have sponsored training workshops throughout the country. Because many existing hemophilia treatment programs are more successful at reaching white middle-class populations, it is especially important that they also develop effective outreach to bring in Black and Latino hemophiliacs for AIDS education.

Address both dimensions of hemophiliacs' concerns: the blood disorder and HIV infection.

AIDS educators not experienced in working with hemophiliacs may assume that AIDS is the paramount concern. In fact, the two are usually inseparable. Dr. Lester Jaffe, director of adolescent medicine at Mt. Sinai Hospital in New York, observed that adolescent hemophiliacs were "often socially immature due to the combination of HIV status and hemophilia." In a program for adolescents with hemophilia, Dr. Jaffe helps young people talk about both conditions and their implications for social and sexual relationships. In order to minimize the denial that the word AIDS evokes in hemophiliacs, Dr. Jaffe labeled these sessions sex education rather than AIDS education.

Discrimination can also encompass both conditions. Dr. Marion Koerper, director of the hemophilia treatment center at the University of California in San Francisco, explained: "If someone walked up to you and said, 'Hello. My name is John, and I have hemophilia,' the immediate reaction would be, 'You must be infected with the AIDS virus.' " AIDS educators need to help people with hemophilia develop strategies for deciding whom to tell about their condition and what to tell them. Like others affected by AIDS, hemophiliacs have the difficult dilemma of balancing personal protection against discrimination and disease prevention. Supportive counselors can play an important role in resolving this dilemma.

Develop peer support groups to help hemophiliacs cope with the threat of HIV infection.

Growing research evidence demonstrates that peer groups can play an important role in chronic disease management. They are especially helpful for adolescents. Both hemophiliacs and their families benefit from opportunities to vent feelings, exchange coping strategies, and discuss problems. The National Hemophilia Foundation and many medical centers already sponsor such support groups. Adding AIDS prevention to their agenda can help many families to better understand and cope with this threat.

Involve family members in AIDS education.

Hemophilia, like any chronic disease, affects the whole family of the affected person. Issues that can arise in regard to either hemophilia or HIV include—

- parents' fears for their children's survival, leading to overprotection or undue restrictions;
- resentment on the part of siblings and family members;
- difficulties in making decisions about reproduction, especially in the face of the double threat of a genetic disorder and perinatal transmission of HIV infection;
- discrimination by schools, employers, neighbors, and others;
- problems in making decisions about sexual activities between hemophiliacs and their partners.

By developing programs that include hemophiliacs and their parents, sex partners, or other significant people, educators can help couples and families consider these issues. Support groups, videos and written materials, and ongoing family counseling are among the techniques that can be used for families.

Develop public education campaigns about hemophilia.

Many of the school discrimination cases against children with AIDS or HIV infection have been aimed at hemophiliacs. The public misperception that hemophiliacs are likely to bleed profusely often contributes to the hysteria. By helping the public at large to gain a more accurate understanding of this blood disorder, at least some of this discrimination may be prevented.

CHAPTER THIRTEEN

Homeless People

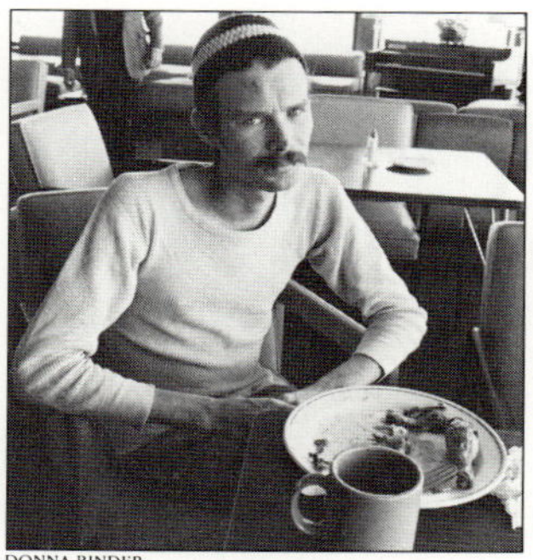

DONNA BINDER

It is estimated that between 300,000 and 3 million Americans are homeless—the uncertainty of the numbers reflects both the lack of reliable data on this problem and the political controversy over the scope and causes of homelessness. In fact, homeless people include a diverse cross-section of populations: mentally ill people released from institutions; youth who have run away or been sent away from their homes; women and children forced out by arson, inadequate income, and housing shortages; and alcohol and substance abusers.

Extent of AIDS and HIV Among the Homeless

How does HIV infection threaten homeless people? Although national data are lacking, a closer look at New York City, where more people are homeless and more have AIDS than anywhere else in the United States, provides a grim portrait of the problem that can be expected in other urban areas as homelessness and HIV infection continue to spread.

- *Doctors who work with homeless people in New York City estimate that by mid-1988, 15% to 20% of the 10,000 residents of shelters for single people were already infected with HIV.*

About 1,000 already have symptoms that would lead to a diagnosis of AIDS. It is estimated that at least 5,000 people with AIDS in New York City are without a home.

- Drug use is common among shelter residents. Surveys suggest that 15% to 30% of those living in New York City shelters for single people are currently using IV drugs. Others have used IV drugs in the past. Cocaine use is also prevalent, in both shelters and welfare hotels. Crack users frequently exchange sex for drugs.
- One researcher reported that 50% of the men he interviewed in a Bronx shelter said they had had sex with other men.
- Tuberculosis rates have risen sharply in New York City, up 35% in the two-year period 1985-86. Tuberculosis is particularly common in homeless shelters. A 1985 study at St. Vincent's Hospital in New York City found that 45% of 1,232 shelter residents examined had antibodies to tuberculosis, indicating previous infection, and 5% were actively infected. Tuberculosis and HIV infection seem to be closely related, perhaps contributing to each other.

Together, these conditions make homeless people especially vulnerable to HIV infection. AIDS educators need to work with those serving the homeless to bring prevention messages to this population. These are a few of the AIDS prevention activities that have been carried out in New York City by staff and residents of programs for the homeless:

- A church sponsored an AIDS education session at a pantry and soup kitchen serving the homeless. Fifty-five persons attended and stayed on long after the scheduled workshop.
- A joint union-management training program gave shelter workers information on AIDS, safety precautions to prevent transmission, and resources available for referral.
- Health workers at a shelter for homeless men in the Bronx showed a film on AIDS, then demonstrated techniques for condom use and needle cleaning. Shelter residents asked many questions. Now AIDS educators are producing a video on AIDS prevention with a group of residents from this shelter.
- Paraprofessional case workers in a welfare hotel were given training on AIDS prevention, then asked to lead informal rap groups for residents. These sessions led into free-flowing discussions of sex, drugs, and health.

Recommendations

The following suggestions will help AIDS educators develop effective prevention programs to reach the homeless:

- Educate the leaders and staff of advocacy and service organizations working with homeless people about preventing AIDS and HIV infection.
- Ask advocacy groups for the homeless to train AIDS educators about homelessness and the local shelter system before programs are planned.
- Include homeless people in the planning and delivery of AIDS education programs.
- Organize networks and coalitions that bring together AIDS organizations and groups serving homeless people.
- Educate public officials and citizens regarding the health and social costs of failing to provide adequate housing.
- Address the specific educational needs of various sectors of the homeless population, such as women and children, those with psychiatric illness, veterans, drug users and alcoholics, youth, and gay men.
- Integrate AIDS prevention into existing health and education programs serving the homeless.

CHAPTER FOURTEEN

People with Developmental Disabilities

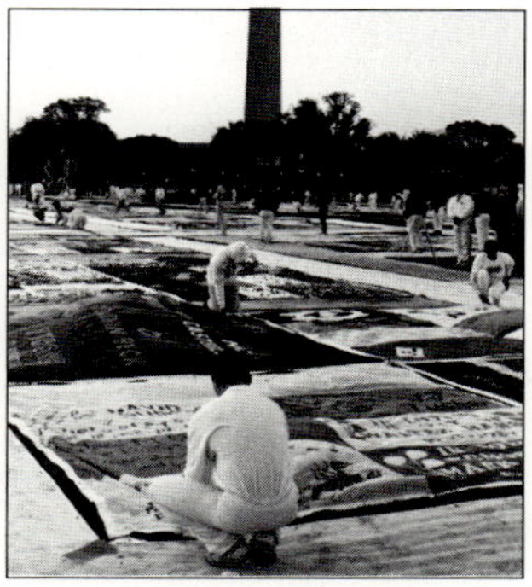

Extent of AIDS Among People with Developmental Disabilities

As AIDS educators and public health officials call for widespread public education about AIDS, people with developmental disabilities have, for the most part, been ignored. This group constitutes between 1% and 5% of the US population, depending on how disability is defined, and includes those with mild to profound retardation.

Education levels among such subgroups vary widely; mildly retarded people can often read at a fourth-grade level, but those who are profoundly retarded cannot understand written materials.

Trends of deinstitutionalization and the increasing number of group homes in the community have meant that many people with developmental disabilities are no longer physically isolated from the larger population. Today, many are allowed greater autonomy than before and therefore need information about sexuality and AIDS. This is particularly true in communities with high prevalence of HIV infection in the overall population, which increases the likelihood that a retarded person's sex partner may be infected.

Many experts believe that because of their cognitive impairment, people with developmental disabilities are at higher risk because they are unlikely to have heard or fully understood much of the information about AIDS that has been transmitted by the media. Further, they are a population that has received little or no basic sex or health education. For all these reasons, people with developmental disabilities present a formidable challenge that AIDS educators can no longer overlook.

Accurate information on the prevalence of AIDS and HIV infection is lacking, but most experts believe that there are as yet only a handful of cases of AIDS among retarded people. One recent seroprevalence study in group homes in New York City found no cases of infection. However, those who work with this population believe that the lack of effective sex and AIDS education puts people with developmental disabilities at risk of HIV infection. Moreover, low current levels of infection make the potential benefits of prevention high.

Problems of AIDS Education for the Developmentally Disabled

Part of the difficulty in implementing AIDS education for this group is that many of the people who administer and develop programs for the developmentally disabled find it difficult to acknowledge that their clients are sexually active. This denial still delays sex education in some agencies and makes it ineffective in others. Some administrators and staff also deny the serious problem of sexual abuse of the developmentally disabled; victims of attacks are at risk for HIV infection.

Still another problem is the lack of expertise in sex education in most staff serving the developmentally disabled. Many workers acknowledge that their patients need education in sexuality, but their own discomfort with the subject, their inadequate skills, and the other pressing demands of their jobs make sex education a low priority.

Even though some states mandate sex education for the staff and residents of group homes, these guidelines are often ignored. Those who do advocate AIDS education and frank information about sexuality and condom use for the developmentally disabled are finding themselves in the same controversial and politically charged situation as those trying to implement AIDS education programs for adolescents.

As in other institutions, homosexual activity is not uncommon in group homes. Homophobia and fears of pregnancy resulting from heterosexual intercourse make some staff ambivalent about their patients' sexual behavior. This ambivalence can contribute to ignoring homosexual behavior.

Although little is known about IV drug use among the retarded, Dr. Susan Pincus, a physician specializing in developmental disability at Montefiore Medical Center in the Bronx, observed that "those who are mentally retarded are unlikely to be capable of the demanding survival skills necessary to maintain oneself as an IV drug addict."

One organization that has developed AIDS and safer-sex education for the developmentally disabled is the Young Adult Institute (YAI) in New York City. YAI is a private, not-for-profit agency serving 1,500 people of all ages and functioning levels through more than 50 programs in the New York City area. It provides a full range of counseling, training, treatment, employment, residential, and family support services.

Because of the needs in its own programs, YAI produced a videotape and training program to educate people with developmental disabilities about AIDS and how to protect themselves. It is aimed primarily at those with mild to moderate retardation.

The goals of the YAI AIDS training program are to ensure that the developmental disabled client will clearly understand—

- what AIDS is;
- how AIDS is spread;
- how people can protect themselves from AIDS;
- how to use a condom;
- how they can develop strategies for resisting social pressure that can put them at risk.

The tape (made by the YAI staff) is explicit, showing both heterosexual and gay couples about to have sex, and all visibly using condoms. It also demonstrates how to put on a condom, using a realistic model of a penis. As expected, its explicitness has caused controversy. YAI maintains that the video does not encourage clients to be sexually active, but that it was designed to help stop the spread of AIDS through teaching proper condom use to consenting adults who have chosen to be sexually active.

Perry Samowitz, YAI's director of education and training (who helped write and produce the AIDS video), noted, "It's explicit because it has to be. People with developmental disabilities don't learn if they don't see it. They can't just listen and really get it." The YAI also developed a staff training manual with specific instructions to be used as a step-by-step guide on how to use the video with clients. The manual includes an intensive follow-up system to help staff provide the individual counseling that is needed to reinforce this information.

In many facilities, staff fears about AIDS transmission are a major obstacle. Teaching staff how HIV infection is and is not spread is a crucial prerequisite for effective AIDS prevention programs. Often, workers' previous experience in protecting themselves against hepatitis B, a common problem for those serving the retarded, can provide a foundation for the skills needed for protection from HIV.

Recommendations

Those working with the developmentally disabled make the following recommendations for AIDS education programs:

- Implement AIDS education for staff, parents, and clients of programs for the developmentally disabled.
- Include parents and staff in the discussion and planning of AIDS education of clients.
- Develop education programs that address the specific learning capabilities of those with varying levels of disability.
- Develop clear AIDS-related agency policies.
- Develop clear policies around sexual behavior, including same-sex behavior, that protect patients against sexual assault while maintaining their right to consensual sex.
- Mandate AIDS education and sex education for all clients, and develop guidelines that specify the content of each program.
- Include experienced sex educators in planning and implementing programs.
- Develop model AIDS education programs for clients that each agency can use or adapt within specific guidelines.
- Organize coalitions and networks that advocate the right of the developmentally disabled to receive adequate health and sexuality education.

A P P E N D I X

Resources

FOR FURTHER READING

Chapter 1: The Social and Political Context of AIDS Education

Altman D: *AIDS in the Mind of America*, Garden City, Anchor, 1986.

Booth W: Another muzzle for AIDS education? *Science* 1987, 238:1036.

Brandt A: *No Magic Bullet: A Social History of Venereal Disease in the U.S. Since 1880,* rev ed, New York, Oxford University Press, 1987.

CDC Update: Acquired immunodeficiency syndrome—United States, 1981-1988. *MMWR* 1989;38:229-236.

Crimp D (ed): *AIDS Cultural Analysis Cultural Activism.* Cambridge, MA: MIT Press, 1988.

Dalton H, Harris S: *AIDS and the Law: A Guide for the Public.* New Haven, Conn, Yale University Press, 1987.

Dondero TJ and HIV Data Analysis Team: Human immunodeficiency virus infection in the United States: a review of current knowledge. *MMWR* 1987(Dec 18 suppl);36(49):5-53.

Feldman D, Johnson T (eds): *The Social Dimensions of AIDS: Method and Theory.* New York, Praeger, 1986.

Fineberg HV: Education to prevent AIDS: prospects and obstacles. *Science* 1988;239:592-596.

Freudenberg N: Historical omissions: a critique of *And the Band Played On. Health/PAC Bulletin* 1988;18(1):16-20.

Institute of Medicine: *Confronting AIDS: Directions For Public Health, Health Care and Research*, Washington, DC, National Academy Press, 1986.

Intergovernmental Health Policy Project: AIDS: A Public Health Challenge. State Issues, Policies and Programs. Washington, DC, George Washington University, 1988.

Kreiger N, Appleman R: *The Politics of AIDS.* Frontline Publications, PO Box 2729, Oakland, CA 94602, 1986.

Lederer R: Origin and spread of AIDS: Is the West responsible? *Covert Action Information Bulletin* 1987; part 1:28:43-54; part 2,29:52-65.

National Academy of Sciences: *Mobilizing Against AIDS*, Cambridge, Mass, Harvard University Press, 1986, and 1988 update.

Osborne J: AIDS, politics and science. *New Engl J Med* 1988;318:444-447.

Patton C: Resistance and the erotic: reclaiming history, setting strategy as we face AIDS. *Radical America* 1987;20(6):68-78.

Patton, C: *Sex and Germs: The Politics of AIDS*, Boston, South End Press, 1985.

Presidential Commission on the Human Immunodeficiency Virus Epidemic: Final commission report. Washington, DC, Government Printing Office, June 24, 1988.

Shilts R: *And the Band Played On*, New York, St Martin's Press, 1987.

Chapter 2: Building Support for AIDS Prevention

Arno PS: The non-profit sector's response to the AIDS epidemic: community-based services in San Francisco. *Am J Public Health* 1986;76:1325-1330.

Carbine ME, Lee P: *AIDS Into the 90s: Strategies for an Integrated Response to the Epidemic*, Washington, DC, National AIDS Network, January 1988.

Frank M: *Management and Organizational Needs Assessment Study of US AIDS Agencies*, Washington, DC, National AIDS Network, 1987.

Judson F, Vernon T: The impact of AIDS on state and local health departments: issues and a few answers. *Am J Public Health* 1988;78:387-393.

Kawata P, Andriote JM: NAN: A national voice for community-based services to persons with AIDS. *Public Health Rep* 1988;103(3):299-304.

Krieger N, Lashof J: AIDS, policy analysis, and the electorate: the role of schools of public health. *Am J Public Health* 1988;78:411-415.

Sundwall D, Bailey D: Meeting the needs of people with AIDS: Local initiatives and federal support. *Public Health Rep* 1988;103(3):293-298.

Chapter 3: Educating for Health: A Framework for AIDS Educators

Asante MR et al: *Handbook of Intercultural Communications*, Beverly Hills, Calif, Sage, 1979.

Bandura A: *Social Learning Theory*, Englewood Cliffs, NJ, Prentice Hall, 1977.

Basch CE: Focus group interview: an underutilized research technique for improving theory and practice in health education. *Health Educ Q* 1987;14(4): 411-448.

Becker M, Joseph J: AIDS and behavior change to reduce risk: a review. *Am J Public Health* 1988;78(4):394-410.

Centers for Disease Control: HIV epidemic and AIDS: trends in knowledge—United States, 1987 and 1988. *MMWR* 1989;38:335-358.

Centers for Disease Control: *Information and Education Plan to Prevent and Control AIDS in the United States*, Washington, DC, Public Health Service, March 1987.

Dawson D, Thornberry O: AIDS knowledge and attitudes for November 1987. *Advancedata* March 16, 1988;151:1-11.

Doak C et al: *Teaching Patients with Low Literacy Skills*, Santa Cruz, Calif, Education Program Associates, 1985.

Fineberg H: Education to prevent AIDS: prospects and obstacles. *Science* 1988;239:592-596.

Green L, Kreuter M, Deeds S, Partridge K: *Health Education Planning: A Diagnostic Approach*, Palo Alto, Calif, Mayfield Publishing, 1980.

Institute of Medicine, National Academy of Sciences: *Health and Behavior: Frontiers of Research in the Biobehavioral Sciences*, Washington, DC, National Academy Press, 1986.

LeFebvre RC, Flora J: Social marketing and public health intervention. *Health Educ Q* 1988;15(3): 299-315.

Rogers E: *Communication Strategies for Family Planning*, New York, The Free Press, 1973.

Siegel K (ed): AIDS education: The public health challenge. *Health Edu Q* 1986;13(4):285-427.

Siegel K, Grodsky P, Herman A: AIDS risk-reduction guidelines: a review and analysis. *Journal of Community Health* 1986;11(4):233-243.

Solomon MZ, DeJong W: Recent sexually transmitted disease prevention efforts and their implications for AIDS health education. *Health Educ Q* 1986; 13(4):301-316.

Turner CF, Miller HG, Moses LE (eds): *AIDS, Sexual Behavior and Intravenous Drug Use*, Washington, DC, National Academy Press, 1989.

Chapter 4: Strategies for AIDS Prevention

Bayer R, Levine C, Wolfe S: HIV antibody screening: an ethical framework for evaluating proposed programs. *JAMA* 1986;256:1768-1774.

Bye L: *Elements of a Comprehensive Community AIDS Prevention Campaign*, San Francisco, Communications Technologies, May 1988. [Communications Technologies, 260 California St, Suite 803, San Francisco, CA 94111].

Cates W, Handsfield H: HIV counseling and testing: does it work? *Am J Public Health* 1988;78:1533-34.

Conant M, Hardy D, Sertnatinger J et al: Condoms prevent transmission of AIDS-associated retrovirus. *JAMA* 1986;255(1):25-27,31.

Echenberg DF: A new strategy to prevent the spread of AIDS among heterosexuals. *JAMA* 1985; 254(15): 2129-2130.

Everett J, Glanz W: *The Condom Book: Essential Guide for Men and Women*. New York, NAL/ Signet, 1987.

Francis DP, Chin J: The prevention of acquired immunodeficiency syndrome in the United States: An objective strategy for medicine, public health, business and the community. *JAMA* 1987; 257(10):1357-66.

Goedert TJ: What is safe sex? Suggested standards linked to testing for HIV. *N Eng J Med* 1987; 316(21): 1339-42.

Goldblum P, Seymour N: Whether to take the test: counseling guidelines. *Focus: A Guide to AIDS Research* 1987;2(5):1-3.

Gostin L, Curran WJ: AIDS screening, confidentiality and the duty to warn. *Am J Public Health* 1987; 77(3):361-365.

Gostin L, Curran WJ: Legal control measures for AIDS: reporting requirements, surveillance, quarantine, and regulation of public meeting places. *Am J Public Health* 1987;77(2):214-218.

Halleron T, Pisanchesi J (eds): *AIDS Information Resource Directory*. New York, American Foundation for AIDS Research, 1988.

Health in the media. *Health Link* 1987;3(2):3-18.

Helquist M: AIDS antibody testing. In: *Working With AIDS: A Resource Guide for Health Professionals*. San Francisco, University of California Regents, 1987, pp. 167-184.

Lee J, Schnee L, Freudenberg N: *Counseling and Education for the Prevention of AIDS: A Curriculum Guide for Training Health and Social Service Workers*, New York, Hunter College, 1988 [425 E 25th St, Box 609, New York, NY 10010].

Meyer KB, Packer SG: Screening for HIV: Can we afford the false positive rate? *New Eng J Med* 1987;317:238-241.

Miller D, Jeffries D, Green J et al: HTLV-III: Should testing ever be routine? *Br Med J* 1986;292(6525): 941-943.

Singer E, Rogers T: Public opinion and AIDS. *AIDS and Public Policy Journal* 1986;1(1):8-13.

Solomon MZ, DeJong W: Preventing AIDS and other STDs through condom promotion: a patient education intervention. *Am J Public Health* 1989;79(4):453-458.

Spain J: *Sexual, Contraceptive and Pregnancy Choice: Counseling Adolescents*, New York, Gardner Press, 1988.

Valdiserri RO et al: The relationship between women's attitudes about condoms and their use: implications for condom promotion programs. *Am J Public Health* 1989;79(4):499-501.

Van Devanter NL, Grisaffi J, Steilen M, et al: Counseling HIV-antibody positive blood donors. *Am J Nurs* 1987;87(8):1026-30.

Weiss EH, Kessel G: Practical skills for health educators on using mass media. *Health Education* (Nov-Dec) 1987:39-41.

Weiss R, Thier S: HIV testing is the answer; what's the question? *New Eng J Med* 1988;319(15):1010.

Chapter 5: Gay and Bisexual Men

Altman D: *The Homosexualization of America*, Boston, Beacon Press, 1983.

Coates TJ, Morin SF, McKusick L: Behavior consequences of AIDS antibody testing among gay men. *JAMA* 1987;258:1889.

Lyter DW et al. The HIV antibody test: Why gay and bisexual men want or do not want to know their results. *Public Health Rep* 1987;102:468-474.

Martin JL: AIDS risk reduction recommendations and sexual behavior patterns among gay men. *Health Educ Q* 1986;13:347-358.

Martin JL: The impact of AIDS on gay male sexual behavior patterns in New York City. *Am J Public Health* 1987;77:578-581.

McCusker J et al: Effects of HIV antibody test knowledge on subsequent sexual behaviors in a cohort of homosexually active men. *Am J Public Health* 1988;78:462-467.

McKusick L, Conant M, Coates TJ: The AIDS epidemic: a model for developing intervention strategies for reducing high-risk behavior in gay men. *Sex Trans Dis* 1985;12:229-234.

Morin SF, Batchelor F: Responding to the psychological crisis of AIDS. *Public Health Reports* 1984;99(1).

Natter J: Safer Sex and AIDS Prevention Policies (unpublished manuscript), New York, Gay Men's Health Crisis, 1986.

Schechter M et al: Patterns of sexual behavior and condom use in a cohort of homosexual men. *Am J Public Health* 1988;78:1535-1538.

Valdiseri R et al: The effect of group education on improving attitudes about AIDS risk reduction. *New York State J Med* 1987;87:272-278.

Winkelstein W et al: The San Francisco men's health study III: Reduction in HIV transmission among homosexual/bisexual men 1982-1986. *Am J Public Health* 1987;77:685-689.

Chapter 6: Intravenous Drug Users

DesJarlais DC, Friedman SR, Hopkins W: Risk reduction for acquired immunodeficiency syndrome among intravenous drug users. *Ann Intern Med* 1985;5(103):755-759.

Friedman SR, DesJarlais DC, Sotheran JL: AIDS health education for intravenous drug users. *Health Educ Q* 1986;13(4):383-393.

Friedman SR et al: AIDS and self-organization among intravenous drug users. *Intl J of Addictions* 1987;22(3):201-219.

Galea R, Lewis B, Baker L (eds): *AIDS and IV Drug Users*, Owings Mills, MD, Rynd Communications, 1988.

Newman R: Methadone treatment: defining and evaluating success. *New Eng J Med* 1987;317:447-450.

Schuster C: Intravenous drug use and AIDS prevention. *Public Health Rep* 1988;103(3):261-266.

Sulima J (ed): *What Every Drug Counselor Should Know About AIDS*, Washington, DC, Manisses Communications, 1987 [Manisses Communications, 1511 K St, NW, Suite 314, Washington, DC 20005].

Chapter 7: African-Americans and Latinos

Amaro H: Considerations for prevention of HIV infection among Hispanic women. *Psychol of Women Q* 1988;12:429-443.

Atkinson D et al: *Counseling American Minorities*, Dubuque, Iowa, William Brown, 1979.

Bouknight RR, Bouknight LG: AIDS in the Black community: focusing on education and the Black male. *NY State J of Med* 1988;88(12):638-641.

Freudenberg N, Lee J, Silver D: How Black and Latino community organizations respond to the AIDS epidemic: A case study in one New York City neighborhood. *AIDS Education and Prevention* 1989;1(1):12-21.

Friedman SR et al: The AIDS epidemic among Blacks and Hispanics. *Milbank Quarterly* 1977;65 (supplement 2):455-499.

Grassroots minority groups fight AIDS. *Health/PAC Bulletin* 1988;18(1):4-10.

Helquist M: AIDS and ethnic communities, in *Working with AIDS: A Resource Guide for Mental Health Professionals*, San Francisco, University of California Regents, 1987, pp 137-156.

Mays V, Cochran S: Acquired immunodeficiency syndrome and Black Americans: special psychosocial issue. *Public Health Repts* 1987;102:224-231.

Mays V, Cochran S: Issues in the perception of AIDS risk and risk reduction activities by Black and Hispanic/Latina women. *Amer Psychologist* 1988;43(11):949-957.

National Council of La Raza: *Who Can Help? Resources and Contacts for Hispanic AIDS Education and Prevention,* Washington, DC, Author, 1988.

Peterson L, Marin G: Issues in the prevention of AIDS in Black and Hispanic men. *Amer Psychologist* 1988;43(11):871-877.

Rogers MF, Williams WW: AIDS in Blacks and Hispanics: implications for prevention. *Issues in Science and Technology* 1987;(3)89-94.

Selik R, Castro K, Pappaioanou M: Racial/ethnic differences in the risk of AIDS in the United States. *Am J Public Health* 1988;78:1539-1545.

Williams LS: AIDS risk reduction: a community health intervention for minority high risk group members. *Health Educ Q* 1986;13(4):407-421.

Chapter 8: Youth

Bennett WH: *AIDS and the Education of Our Children: A Guide for Parents and Teachers*, Washington, DC, US Dept of Education, October 1987.

Black JL: AIDS: preschool and school issues. *J School Health* 1986;3(56):93-95.

Caruso BA, Haig JR: AIDS on campus: a survey of college health service priorities and policies. *J Am Coll Health* 1987;36(1):32-36.

Cates W, Rauh JL: Adolescent sexually transmitted diseases: an expanding problem. *J Adolesc Health Care* 1985;6:257-261.

Centers for Disease Control: Guidelines for effective school health education to prevent the spread of AIDS. *MMWR* 1988;37(suppl S-2):1-14.

DiClemente RJ, Boyer CB, Morales ED: Minorities and AIDS: knowledge, attitudes and misconceptions among Black and Latino adolescents. *Am J Public Health* 1988;78:55-57.

DiClemente RJ, Zorn J, Temoshok L: Adolescents and AIDS: a survey of knowledge, attitudes and beliefs about AIDS in San Francisco. *Am J Public Health* 1986;76:1443-1445.

English A: Adolescents and AIDS: legal and ethical questions multiply. *Youth Law News* 1987; 8(6):1-6.

Haffner D: *AIDS and Adolescents: The Time for Prevention is Now*, Center for Population Options, 1987 [Center for Population Options, 1012 14th St, NW, Washington, DC, 20005].

Hein K: AIDS in adolescents: a rationale for concern. *NY State J of Med* 1987;87:290-295.

Jaffe L, Wortman R: The fear of AIDS guidelines to the counseling and HTLV-III antibody screening of adolescents. *J Adolesc Health Care* 1988;9: 84-86.

Jones EF et al: Teenage pregnancy in developed countries: determinants and policy implications. *Fam Plann Perspect* 1985;17:53-63.

Kegeles SM, Adler NE, Irwin C: Sexually active adolescents and condoms: changes over one year in knowledge, attitudes and use. *Am J Public Health* 1988;78(4);460-461.

Kelling R: *AIDS on the College Campus: ACHA Special Report*, Rockville, MD, American College Health Association, 1986.

Kodama C: *AIDS Education on the College Campus: A Practical Guide*, Berkeley, Calif, UC Berkeley Student Health Service, 1987.

Mantell J, Schinke S: The crisis of AIDS for adolescents: the need for preventive risk-reduction interventions, in Roberts AR (ed): *Crisis Intervention Handbook*, New York, Springer, 1988.

McDermott RJ et al: AIDS awareness and information sources among selected university students. *J Am College Health* 1987;35(5):222-226.

National Coalition of Advocates for Students: *Criteria for Evaluating an AIDS Curriculum*, Boston, National Coalition of Advocates for Students, 1987 [NCAS, 100 Boylston St, 737, Boston, MA 02116].

Price JH: AIDS, the schools, and policy issues. *J School Health* 1986;56(4):137-140.

Quackenbush M, Sargent P: *Teaching AIDS: A Resource Guide,* Santa Cruz, Calif, ETR Associates, 1986 [ETR Associates, 1700 Mission St, Suite 203, Santa Cruz, CA 95061].

Remafedi G: Homosexual youth: a challenge to contemporary society. *JAMA* 1987;258(2):222-225.

Remafedi G: Male homosexuality: the adolescent's perspective. *Pediatrics* 1987;79:326-330.

Report of the Surgeon General's Workshop on Children with HIV Infection and Their Families, Washington, DC, US Dept of Health and Human Services, 1987.

Schinazi R, Nahmias A: *AIDS in Children, Adolescents and Heterosexuals: An Interdisciplinary Perspective,* New York, Elsevier Publishing, 1988.

Strunin L, Hingson R: Acquired immunodeficiency syndrome and adolescents: knowledge, beliefs, attitudes and behaviors. *Pediatrics* 1987;79: 825-828.

Chapter 9: Women

Donovan P: AIDS and family planning clinics: confronting the crisis. *Fam Plann Perspect* 1987;19(3):111-14,138.

Dryfoos JG: Contraceptive use, pregnancy intentions and pregnancy outcome among US women. *Fam Plann Perspect* 1982;14:18-81.

Guinan ME, Hardy A: Epidemiology of AIDS in women in the United States: 1981 through 1986. *JAMA* 1987;257:2039-2042.

Helquist M: The impact of AIDS on women, in *Working With AIDS: A Resource Guide for Mental Health Professionals,* San Francisco, University of California Regents, 1987, pp 119-138.

Mantell J, Akabar S, Schintene S: Women and AIDS prevention. *Journal of Primary Prevention* [in press].

Patton C, Kelly J: *Making It: A Woman's Guide to Sex in the Age of AIDS,* Ithaca, NY, Firebrand Books, 1987 [Firebrand Books, 141 Commons, Ithaca, NY 14850].

Richardson D: *Women and AIDS,* New York, Muthaven, 1988.

Rosenberg M, Weiner J: Prostitutes and AIDS: a health department priority? *Am J Public Health* 1988;78:418-423.

Sachs BP, Tuomala R, Frigoletto F: Acquired immunodeficiency syndrome: suggested protocol for counseling and screening in pregnancy. *Obstet Gynecol* 1987;70 (3 part 1):408-411.

Worth D, Rodriguez R: Latina women and AIDS. *SEICUS Report* 1987;Jan/Feb:5-7.

Chapter 10: Workers

AIDS in the Workplace, special issue of *EAP Digest* 1988; May/June.

Banta WF: *AIDS in the Workplace: Legal Questions and Practical Answers,* Lexington, ME, Lexington Books, 1987.

Bauman LJ, Abernath J: Health educators in the workplace: helping companies respond to the AIDS crisis. *Health Educ Q* 1986;13(4):395-406.

Emery A, Puckett S: *Managing AIDS in the Workplace,* San Francisco, San Francisco AIDS Foundation, 1988.

Feurer D: AIDS at work: fighting the fear. *Training* 1987;(June)61-71.

Gerbert B et al: Fear of AIDS: issues for health professional education. *AIDS Education and Prevention* 1989;1(1):39-52.

Krapfl M: As AIDS hysteria spreads so does need for cool-headed education. *Occup Health Saf* 1986;55(4):20-29.

Marcus R, CDC Cooperative Needlestick Surveillance Group: Surveillance of health care workers exposed to blood from patients infected with HIV. *New Eng J Med* 1988;319(17):1118.

Masi D: AIDS in the workplace: what can be done. *Personnel* 1987;(July)57-60.

Mason JM: Statement on the development of guidelines for the prevention of AIDS transmission in the workplace. *Public Health Rep* 1986;1(101): 6-8.

New York Business Group on Health: *AIDS and the Employer: Guidelines for Managing AIDS in the Workplace.* New York, Business Group on Health, 1986 [Business Group on Health, 622 Third Ave, New York, NY 10017].

O'Donnell L, O'Donnell C: Hospital workers and AIDS: effect of inservice education on knowledge and perceived risks and stresses. *NY State J Med* 1987;87:278-280.

Searle ES: Knowledge, attitudes and behavior of health professionals in relation to AIDS. *Lancet* 1987;8253(1):26-28.

Service Employees International Union: *The AIDS Book: Information for Workers* (1987 suppl), Washington, DC, Service Employees International Union [SEIU, 1313 L St, NW, Washington, DC 20005].

Valenti WM, Angrella JP: Survey of hospital personnel on the understanding of AIDS. *Am J Infection Control* 1986;14:60-63.

Wertz D et al: Knowledge and attitudes of AIDS health care providers before and after education programs. *Public Health Reports* 1987;102(3): 248-254.

Chapter 11: Prisoners

Hammett TM: *AIDS in Correctional Facilities: Issues and Options.* US Dept of Justice/National Institute of Justice, April 1986 (third ed., April 1988).

Hammett TM: *Update 1988: AIDS in Correctional Facilities.* US Dept of Justice/National Institute of Justice, January 1989.

Jones BS, Philyaw JE: *Correctional Facilities: Toward a Strategy (Going Into Prison with AIDS Education).* National AIDS Network Multi-Cultural NOTES on AIDS Education and Service, 1-3 Nov. 1987.

Krupp LB, Gelberg EA, Wormser G: Prisoners as medical patients. *Am J Public Health* 1987;77(7).

Ortega N: AIDS policies tested in Alabama prison case. *NPP Journal* 1980;16:8-9.

Potler C: *AIDS in Prison: A Crisis in New York State Corrections,* New York, Correctional Association of New York, 1988.

Vaid U: AIDS among prisoners: facts, myths and problems. In: *AIDS/Law Sourcebook,* New Haven, Conn, Yale University Press, 1987.

Vaid U: AIDS in prisons. In: *AIDS Legal Guide: A Professional Resource on AIDS-Related Legal Issues and Discrimination.* New York, Lambda Legal Defense and Education Fund, 1987 [666 Broadway, New York, NY 10011].

Chapter 12: People with Hemophilia and Other Blood Disorders

Hargraves M, Jason J, Chorba T et al: Hemophiliac patients' knowledge and educational needs concerning acquired immunodeficiency syndrome. *Am J Hematol* 1987;26(2):115-24.

Sussman R: People with hemophilia: psychosocial factors, in Moffat B et al (eds): *AIDS: A Self-Care Manual,* Los Angeles, AIDS Project Los Angeles, 1987.

Chapter 13: Homeless People

Haus A (ed): *Working with Homeless People: A Guide for Staff and Volunteers,* New York, Columbia University Community Services, 1988 [Columbia University Community Services, 635 W 115th St, New York, NY 10025].

Chapter 14: People with Developmental Disabilities

Chamberlain A et al: Issues in fertility control for mentally retarded female adolescents. *Pediatrics* 1984;73(4):445-450.

Edgerton RB: Alcohol and drug use by mentally retarded adults. *Am J Mental Deficiency* 1986; 90(6):602-609.

Kastner TA, Hickman ML, Bellehumeur D: The provision of services to persons with mental retardation and subsequent infection with human immunodeficiency virus (HIV). *Am J Public Health* 1989;79(4):491-494.

Levy P: *Staff and Client Training Curriculum for HIV.* New York: Young Adult Institute, 1987.

Pincus S: Sexuality in the mentally retarded patient. *Am Family Practitioner* 1988;37(2):319-323.

Simonds JF: Sexual behaviors in retarded children and adolescents. *J Develop Beh Ped* 1980;1(4): 173-179.

Publications on People with AIDS

Callen M (ed): *Surviving and Thriving With AIDS: Hints for the Newly Diagnosed.* New York, People With AIDS Coalition Inc, vol I, 1987;vol II, 1988.

Delaney M, Goldblum P: *Strategies for Survival: A Gay Men's Health Manual for the Age of AIDS,* New York, St Martin's Press, 1987.

Lambda Legal Defense and Education Fund: *Living with AIDS: A Guide to the Legal Problems of People with AIDS,* New York, Lambda, 1987.

Martelli L: *When Someone You Know Has AIDS: A Practical Guide.* New York, Crown Publishers, 1987.

Moffat B, Spiegel J et al: *AIDS: A Self-Care Manual,* Los Angeles, AIDS Project Los Angeles, 1987.

ORGANIZATIONS

General AIDS Education and Advocacy

National AIDS Network
1012 14th St, NW, Suite 601
Washington, DC 20005
(202) 347-0390

Support organization for community groups, clinics, and education projects. Provides technical assistance, referral services, and grants to member groups.

National AIDS Information Clearinghouse
PO Box 6003
Rockville, MD 20850
(301) 762-5111

Sponsored by federal Centers for Disease Control (CDC). Accesses data bases listing local and national AIDS organizations and educational materials. Offers information and referral for AIDS program managers and health professionals. Includes Spanish bilingual reference specialist. Distributes federal AIDS publications (available directly from [800] 458-5231).

National AIDS Hotline
(24 hours a day, 7 days a week)
(800) 342-AIDS

Operated by American Social Health Association for CDC. Offers information and referrals on AIDS prevention and services for those with AIDS.

AIDS Coalition to Network, Organize and Win (ACT NOW)
2300 Market St, Suite 87
San Francisco, CA 94114

National network of local AIDS activist groups doing research, advocacy, and direct action for release of AIDS treatments, full funding of AIDS services and education, and against AIDS-related discrimination and misinformation. Provides information on problems with governmental and private responses to AIDS, based on the perspectives of the affected communities.

American Foundation for AIDS Research (AmFAR)
40 West 57th St, Suite 406
New York, NY 10019
(212) 719-0033

Publishes AIDS Information Resources Directory, listing broad variety of AIDS education materials and films, with reviews by expert panelists.

AIDS Education Office
American Red Cross
1730 D St, NW
Washington, DC 20006
(202) 639-3223

Provides training and educational materials on AIDS for use in schools, workplaces, black and Latino communities, and for the general public.

Sex Information and Education Council of the United States (SIECUS)
32 Washington Pl
New York, NY 10003
(212) 673-3850

Offers annotated bibliography on AIDS education. Has large library, including many sex education curricula, and speakers bureau on sex education.

National Center for Health Education
30 E 29th St
New York, NY 10016
(212) 689-1886

Offers elementary school health curriculum including major AIDS component.

Education Department
Planned Parenthood Federation of America
810 Seventh Ave
New York, NY 10019
(212) 603-4626

Provides clearinghouse and data bases on sexuality and AIDS education curricula, publications, and films.

Fund for Human Dignity
666 Broadway
New York, NY 10012
(212) 529-1600

Operates AIDS Hotline, staffed by lesbians and gay men, and particularly attuned to the issues of gay individuals concerning AIDS.

Local AIDS Service Organizations

Of the many local AIDS service organizations, the following are especially notable for their wide array of educational materials and information on many aspects of AIDS. Each provides comprehensive educational programs offering publications, videos, and speakers. (San Francisco AIDS Foundation offers a wide-ranging *AIDS Educator Catalog* listing brochures, posters, books, multimedia campaigns, and videos.) These organizations also provide counseling, support groups, and specialized services for those with AIDS.

Gay Men's Health Crisis (GMHC)
129 W 20th St
New York, NY 10011
(212) 807-3103
(212) 807-6655 (hotline)

AIDS Project Los Angeles
3670 Wilshire Blvd, Suite 300
Los Angeles, CA 90010
(213) 380-2000

San Francisco AIDS Foundation
333 Valencia St, 4th Floor
San Francisco, CA 94103
(415) 861-3397

Health Education Resource Organization (HERO)
101 W Read St, Suite 812
Baltimore, MD 21201
(301) 685-1180

AIDS Treatment Information

American Foundation for AIDS Research (AmFAR)
40 W 57th St, Suite 406
New York, NY 10019
(212) 719-0033

Publishes *Directory of Experimental Treatments* for AIDS and ARC, periodically updated, with information on clinical trials.

AIDS Treatment News
PO Box 411256
San Francisco, CA 94141
(415) 282-0110

Weekly newsletter of new developments in a wide range of AIDS treatment approaches.

Project Inform
25 Taylor St, Room 618
San Francisco, CA 94102
(800) 822-7422

Clearinghouse on experimental AIDS treatments. Offers phone updates and periodic newsletter.

Health Education AIDS Liaison (HEAL)
PO Box 1103
New York, NY 10013
(212) 674-HOPE

Distributes information by phone and publications on alternative treatments for people with HIV, ARC, and AIDS. Also has a weekly support group for people using alternative treatments.

People with AIDS, ARC, and HIV

National Association of People With AIDS
2025 "I" St, NW, Suite 415
Washington, DC 20006
(202) 429-2856

Network of local groups organized by and for people with AIDS. Provides information and referrals on services, treatments, and rights of people with AIDS and advocates their concerns.

Body Positive
263A W 19th St, Room 107
New York, NY 10011
(212) 633-1782

Offers publications, counseling, advocacy, and referrals for HIV-antibody-positive people.

Legal Issues

Lambda Legal Defense and Education Fund
666 Broadway
New York, NY 10012
(212) 995-8585

Nonprofit law firm offering publications on legal rights of people with AIDS. Files test case suits on discrimination against gay people and those with AIDS.

AIDS Civil Rights Project
National Gay Rights Advocates
8389 Santa Monica Blvd, Suite 202
Los Angeles, CA 90069
(213) 650-6200

Nonprofit law firm handling test cases on discrimination against gay people and people with AIDS. Offers technical assistance to lawyers handling similar cases. Distributes publications on AIDS-related discrimination and corporate policies on AIDS.

AIDS Project
American Civil Liberties Union Foundation
132 W 43rd St
New York, NY 10036
(212) 944-9800

Offers publications with legal and policy analyses of AIDS civil liberties issues. Handles test cases.

Drug Abuse and AIDS

Association for Drug Abuse Prevention and Treatment (ADAPT)
85 Bergen St
Brooklyn, NY 11201
(718) 834-9585

Organization of recovering addicts doing street education on AIDS prevention in New York City, and advocating government support of AIDS education and drug treatment for IV drug users. Operates speakers' bureau and offers training for AIDS service volunteers. Distributes AIDS prevention brochures for IV drug users.

Substance Abuse and AIDS Information Service
Department of Substance Abuse
American Medical Association
535 N Dearborn
Chicago, IL 60610
(312) 645-5000

Publishes free monthly newsletter on AIDS and drug abuse and distributes paper giving overview of prevention approaches for IV drug users.

AIDS Office
Haight Ashbury Free Medical Clinic
529 Clayton St
San Francisco, CA 94117
(415) 621-2014

Offers simple-language, bilingual comic books and brochures on AIDS prevention for IV drug users; also brochures and a video on health maintenance for HIV-positive IV drug users.

People with Hemophilia and AIDS

National Hemophilia Foundation
110 Greene St, Room 406
New York, NY 10012
(212) 219-8180

Distributes publications on hemophilia and AIDS, including specific ones for women and adolescents. Accesses data base on local groups and publications. Offers provider workshops on AIDS. Performs research on AIDS and hemophilia. Does advocacy for people with hemophilia, including fighting discrimination.

People of Color and AIDS

Office of Minority Affairs
National AIDS Network (NAN)
2033 M St, NW, Suite 800
Washington, DC 20003
(202) 293-2437

Provides technical assistance to local AIDS service providers. Operates a project on AIDS and women of color. Publishes bimonthly newsletter. Does advocacy on AIDS and people of color with federal and private organizations.

National Minority AIDS Council
714 G St, SE
PO Box 28574
Washington, DC 20003
(202) 544-1076

Provides technical assistance, leadership training, and help in establishing volunteer programs in communities of color. Also offers publications and referrals, and does advocacy on concerns of people of color.

Multicultural Prevention Resources
1540 Market St, Suite 320
San Francisco, CA 94102
(415) 861-2142

Provides training and technical assistance to AIDS education projects. Offers publications on AIDS for people of color in several languages.

Association of Asian/Pacific Community Health Organizations
310 8th St, Suite 210
Oakland, CA 94607
(415) 272-9536

Provides information and education on health programs for Asian/Pacific peoples.

National Coalition of Hispanic Health and Human Services Organizations (COSSMHO)
1030 15th St, NW, Suite 1053
Washington, DC 20005
(202) 371-2100
(800) AIDS-123 (hotline)

Membership organization of professionals. Operates technical assistance hotline for Hispanic educators. Provides technical assistance for AIDS education programs serving Hispanic women and youth. Offers curriculum for trainers of parents educating children about AIDS. Distributes policy paper on AIDS and Hispanics.

National Native American AIDS Prevention Center
5266 Boyd Ave
Oakland, CA 94618
(415) 654-2093

Network of Native American AIDS activists. Provides training and technical assistance to local groups.

People of Color Against AIDS Network
105 14th St, Suite 2D
Seattle, WA 98128
(206) 332-7061

Offers educational materials. Sponsors conferences. Emphasizes community organizing approach to AIDS.

National Coalition of Black Lesbians and Gays
19641 West Seven Mile
Detroit, MI 48219
(313) 537-0484

Network of local groups. Offers speakers, workshop facilitators, and publications (including a training manual for AIDS educators) on AIDS and sexuality for black gay men and lesbians.

Haitian Women's Program
American Friends Service Committee
15 Rutherford Pl
New York, NY 10003
(212) 598-0965

Offers health education curriculum (including AIDS) for Haitians. Distributes AIDS prevention booklet and video in Creole and English. Does advocacy on Haitian concerns. Offers referral to other Haitian groups.

Women and AIDS

National Resource Center on Women and AIDS
Center for Women Policy Studies
2000 P St, NW, Suite 508
Washington, DC 20036
(202) 872-1770

Publishes resource guide on women and AIDS (prevention and treatment) and a policy paper. Provides technical assistance to women's organizations doing AIDS education. Has speakers' bureau. Provides referrals to local groups.

National Women's Health Network
1325 G St, NW, Lower Level
Washington, DC 20005
(202) 347-1140

Offers publications (including workshop kit for educators) and referrals on women and AIDS.

Women and AIDS Resource Network (WARN)
PO Box 020525
Brooklyn, NY 11202
(718) 596-6007

Provides information and support, and does advocacy, for women at risk for AIDS in the New York City area. Offers publications.

California Prostitutes Education Project (CALPEP)
333 Valencia, 2nd Floor
San Francisco, CA 94103
(415) 558-0450

Offers training (nationwide) for prostitute education projects. Publishes manual for prostitute educators. Project of COYOTE and National Task Force on Prostitution, which also do advocacy and publish policy recommendations on prostitutes and AIDS.

Youth and AIDS

Hetrick-Martin Institute
(Institute for the Protection of Lesbian and Gay Youth)
401 West St
New York, NY 10014
(212) 633-8920

Provides technical assistance and speakers on AIDS prevention, both for lesbian/gay and heterosexual youth, also for professionals working with youth. Offers AIDS prevention publications aimed at lesbian/gay youth. Provides daytime phone counseling for lesbian/gay youth.

National Coalition of Advocates for Students
100 Boylston St, Suite 737
Boston, MA 02116
(617) 357-8507

Distributes publications on school curricula on AIDS (for parents and teachers). Does advocacy for AIDS education with school support professionals.

AIDS Education
American College Health Association
1300 Piccard Drive, Suite 200
Rockville, MD 20850
(301) 963-1100

Offers AIDS workshops for health educators and resident advisors. Distributes publications for educators and students.

Workers and AIDS

National Leadership Coalition on AIDS
1150 17th St, NW, Suite 202
Washington, DC 20036
(202) 429-0930

Coalition which includes corporate leaders concerned about AIDS. Distributes materials on workplace education and AIDS policies.

San Francisco AIDS Foundation
333 Valencia St, 4th Floor
San Francisco, CA 94103
(415) 861-3397

Distributes videos, booklets, and manuals on workplace AIDS education.

American Hospital Association
840 North Lake Shore Dr
Chicago, IL 60611
(312) 280-6000

Distributes pamphlets and videos for health workers and managers. Recommends AIDS-related policies.

Service Employees International Union (SEIU)
1313 L St, NW
Washington, DC 20005
(202) 898-3386

Offers publications on AIDS and workplace issues.

Prisoners and AIDS

AIDS Clearinghouse
National Institute of Justice
National Criminal Justice Reference Service
Box 6000
Rockville, MD 20850
(301) 251-5500

Clearinghouse on AIDS policies and programs in correctional institutions. Publishes reports on AIDS in prisons.

American Correctional Health Services Association
5530 Wisconsin Ave, NW, Suite 745
Washington, DC 20815
(301) 652-1172

Professional organization of health workers in prisons. Issues policy papers on AIDS in prisons.

National Prison Project
American Civil Liberties Union
1616 P St, NW
Washington, DC 20036
(202) 331-0500

Represents inmates challenging prison policies and programs. Serves as network for prison advocates working on AIDS issues. Publishes newsletter on prisoners' rights.

National Lawyers Guild AIDS Network
558 Capp St
San Francisco, CA 94110
(415) 824-8884

Network of prison advocates concerned about AIDS issues.

Homeless People and AIDS

Coalition for the Homeless
105 E 22nd St
New York, NY 10010
(212) 460-8110

Advocacy organization with New York City focus but national interests. Extensive experience in advocating for homeless people with AIDS.

Legal Action Center for the Homeless
220 E 4th St
New York, NY 10003
(212) 529-4240

Represents homeless people, including those with AIDS.

Caucus to House Homeless People with AIDS
AIDS Coalition to Unleash Power (ACT UP)
496A Hudson St, Suite G4
New York, NY 10014
(212) 533-8888

Advocates policies to obtain housing for homeless people with AIDS in New York City. Distributes literature on problems and proposed solutions.

People with Developmental Disabilities and AIDS

Young Adult Institute
460 W 34th St
New York, NY 10001
(212) 563-7474

Distributes training video and manual on AIDS for staff of programs serving developmentally disabled.

Center for AIDS Prevention Education
c/o Polaris Research and Development
China Basin, Suite 6600
185 Berry St
San Francisco, CA 94107
(415) 777-3229

Distributes AIDS training package developed for developmentally disabled and those with learning disabilities.

About the author

Nicholas Freudenberg is Professor and Director of the program in Community Health Education at Hunter College/City University of New York. He also directs the Hunter College Center for Community Action to Prevent AIDS, which provides training and consultation on AIDS prevention to community organizations in New York City. Freudenberg chairs the APHA Society of Public Health Education Task Force on AIDS Education. He holds an MPH and a DrPH from Columbia University School of Public Health.

Photography:

Donna Binder, Impact Visuals: *Pages 107, 125, 199*

Gay Men's Health Crisis: *Pages 1, 19, 63*

Doug Hinckle, Washington Blade, Inc.: *Pages iii, 35, 151, 167, 177, 187, 195, 201*

John Long, Longshots: *Cover*

Ellen B. Neipris, Impact Visuals: *Page vii*

C. T. Wemple, Impact Visuals: *Page 139*